THE REGIONAL MEDICAL CAMPUS

A Resource for Faculty, Staff and Learners

December 2018

Dear Mack—
    Thanks for being such a strong champion of FCM scholarship!
        — Mike

by Michael P. Flanagan, M.D., FAAFP

The Regional Medical Campus, a Resource for Faculty, Staff and Learners

Library of Congress Cataloging-in-Publication Data

Names: Flanagan, Michael P., editor.
Title: The regional medical campus / [edited by] Michael P. Flanagan.
Description: Ocala, Florida : Atlantic Publishing Group, Inc., [2018] |
 Includes bibliographical references and index.
Identifiers: LCCN 2018040651 (print) | LCCN 2018041338 (ebook) | ISBN
 9781620234945 (ebook) | ISBN 9781620234938 (pbk.) | ISBN 1620234939
 (pbk.)
Subjects: | MESH: Schools, Medical--organization & administration |
 Education, Premedical--organization & administration | Education,
 Medical--organization & administration | United States | Canada
Classification: LCC R735 (ebook) | LCC R735 (print) | NLM W 19 AA1 | DDC
 610.71/1--dc23
LC record available at https://lccn.loc.gov/2018040651

Printed in the United States

PROJECT MANAGER: Danielle Lieneman • dlieneman@atlantic-pub.com
INTERIOR LAYOUT, COVER & JACKET DESIGN: Antoinette D'Amore • addesign@videotron.ca

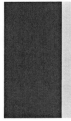

What Faculty, Staff and Learners at Regional Medical Campuses Are Saying

Paula Termuhlen, MD:

The Regional Medical Campus: A Resource for Faculty, Staff and Learners is a one-stop shopping compendium of all things "regional campus". This will serve as an important resource for the growth and development of regional campuses across North America. Together with the new *Journal of Regional Medical Campuses*, this resource provides a voice for all of us who are committed to medical education using the regional campus model and shines a light on the expertise we can provide for those who wish to join us in the journey!

> **Paula M. Termuhlen, M.D.,** Professor of Surgery
> Editor-in-Chief, *The Journal of Regional Medical Campuses*
> Regional Campus Dean, University of Minnesota Medical School, Duluth Campus

Gerry Cooper, MD:

Writer William Gibson has said that the future is here, it's just not widely distributed yet. Regional Medical Campuses (RMCs) are a big part of medical education's future and despite their being found throughout North America, scholarly work regarding RMCs is a recent phenomenon. This book is a major step forward in assembling and distributing the insights of some of RMCs foremost thinkers and academics. It is an inspiring read for medical educators and all who value innovation.

> **Gerry Cooper, M.D.,** Professor of Psychiatry
> Associate Dean, Windsor Campus
> Schulich School of Medicine & Dentistry, Western University
> Ontario, Canada

⁂

John McCarthy, MD:

The Association of American Medical Colleges's (AAMC) Group on Regional Medical Campuses (GRMC) has been highly engaged in and supportive of developing this guide for students, campuses, and regional leadership. The unique and diverse strengths of regional campuses have advanced both undergraduate and graduate medical education across the continent over the last 50 years. Codifying the international diversity of our regional medical campuses through this book will add value to anyone invested in regional or central campus medical education.

> **John McCarthy, M.D.,** Clinical Professor of Family Medicine
> Chair, *Group on Regional Medical Campuses,*
> Association of American Medical Colleges
> Assistant Dean for Rural Affairs, University of Washington
> School of Medicine-Gonzaga Campus

⁂

Kevin Black, MD:

In the absence of change, there is no opportunity for innovation. Within medical education, there is no better opportunity for innovation than a regional medical campus. This book serves as a foundational spark to accelerate change that will enhance the learning experiences of the next generation of physicians. The lessons learned will benefit students and faculty across all types of campuses for years to come.

> **Kevin Black, M.D.**
> C. McCollister Evarts Chair, Department of Orthopaedics and Rehabilitation, Milton S. Hershey Medical Center
> Vice Dean, University Park Regional Campus,
> Penn State College of Medicine

Eric Leemis, MHA:

As an administrator, it is important to understand your operating model relative to others in the same industry. *The Regional Medical Campus: A Resource for Faculty, Staff and Learners* provides a wealth of information on how regional campuses are organized, governed, and funded. I would encourage anyone involved in the delivery of medical education to review this excellent resource for insights into the regional campus model.

> **Eric Leemis, MHA**
> Director, Finance and Administration
> University of Arkansas for Medical Sciences
> Northwest Regional Campus

Peter Nalin, MD:

Whether optimizing an existing regional medical campus, or adding new regional campuses, this practical resource delivers something for everyone associated with the wonderful world of regional medical education.

> **Peter M. Nalin, M.D., FAAFP**
> Associate Vice President in University Clinical Affairs
> Senior Associate Dean for Education Expansion
> Associate Dean & Interim Director, Bloomington
> Regional Campus
> Indiana University School of Medicine

Terry Wolpaw MD, MHPE:

Regional medical campuses make a critical contribution to the dissemination of educational opportunities and ideas across a variety of geographic and healthcare settings. Today they have an ever increasing role as an important locus of innovation in our efforts to accelerate change in medical education. By embracing the opportunity for innovation and collaborating to enhance promising initiatives, regional medical campuses bring important insights to the imperative of better aligning medical education with the skills needed in the continuously evolving healthcare settings where our students will eventually practice.

> **Terry Wolpaw, M.D., MHPE**
> Vice Dean for Educational Affairs
> Penn State College of Medicine

Kathryn Martin, PhD, MPA, MPA:

Accepting the charge to create a Regional Medical Center takes guts, with little to no map, footprint, or instruction manual to follow. This book will provide readers with a glimpse of the worlds where we have created our regional campuses. It provides brief overviews of process, do's and don'ts, and challenges that were overcome through our commitment to medicine, passion for teaching, and hard work to accomplish a novel event. Read on and learn much — then share your stories with us. In other words, "see one, do one, teach one."

> **Kathryn Martin, Ph.D., MPA, MPA,**
> Associate Dean for Regional Campus Development
> Medical College of Georgia at Augusta University

Audreanna James (US Medical Student)

As a third year medical student, I found this book to have useful information, such as developing a student-run clinic and promoting a nutrition curriculum. Having such a resource will allow medical students to incorporate new programing at their own Regional Medical Campus and provide a reference when making changes. Students can use this book to gain insight and it will provide contacts should they have questions.

> **Audreanna James,** Third-Year Medical Student
> Statewide Campus Site Representative
> West Virginia School of Osteopathic Medicine, Class of 2019
> West Virginia University Eastern Campus

Samuel Bergeron (Canadian Medical Student)

As a medical student leader from a regional campus, I can easily relate to the builders who came before me and made a tangible difference in the healthcare system of my community. Reading this book will help to show you where Regional Medical Campuses come from, to better understand where we are going and to help shape the agents of change in the generations to come.

> **Samuel Bergeron,** Fourth-Year Medical Student
> Université de Montréal, Campus Mauricie, Class of 2018
> President of the Fédération médicale étudiante du Québec, representing the 4,200 medical students of Quebec province.

Editor in Chief

Michael P. Flanagan, M.D., FAAFP
Assistant Dean for Student Affairs
Professor and Vice-Chair of Family and Community Medicine
Penn State College of Medicine, University Park Campus

Contributing Editors

Kristen M. Grine, D.O.
Assistant Professor of Family and Community Medicine
Penn State College of Medicine, University Park Campus

Christopher R. Heron, M.D.
Assistant Professor of Family and Community Medicine
Penn State College of Medicine, University Park Campus

E. Eugene Marsh, M.D.
Founding Senior Associate Dean
Professor of Neurology and Master Educator
Penn State College of Medicine, University Park Campus

Mark B. Stephens, M.D., MS, FAAFP
Professor of Family and Community Medicine
Associate Vice-Chair for Research
Penn State College of Medicine, University Park Campus

Jeffrey G. Wong, M.D.
Associate Dean for Education
Professor of Medicine
Penn State College of Medicine, University Park Campus

Dedication

This book is dedicated to Bill and Honora Jaffe,
whose consistent generosity through the
Jaffe Family Endowment for
Family and Community Medicine
at the Penn State College of Medicine,
has helped to make this project possible.

Acknowledgements

This book would not have been possible without the support and contributions of several dedicated individuals. First, I would like to thank the members of the *Group on Regional Medical Campuses* (GRMC) at the Association of American Medical Colleges (AAMC) for your thoughtful contributions to "our" book. I am also grateful to our GRMC leaders, Lanita Carter, Ph.D. and John McCarthy, M.D., for consistently providing a space to promote this project at GRMC meetings. Thanks also goes to Ethan Kendrick, Stephen McKenzie, and Kate McOwen at the AAMC for their encouraging advice and gentle guidance during the past three years.

Next I need to thank my five faculty co-editors for their steadfast dedication to the editing assignments that I repeatedly sent their way. Specifically, Gene Marsh, M.D. for his reliable wisdom and for composing the Foreword; Jeff Wong, M.D. and Kristen Grine, D.O. for their consistent encouragement along the way; Mark Stephens, M.D. for his unbridled enthusiasm; and Kit Heron, M.D. for his exceptional IT expertise. I also want to thank my office nurse, Lynne Corl, for being a positive force of optimism on a daily basis.

Gratitude is due, as well, to my former Department Chair and mentor, Jim Herman, M.D., who encouraged me early in my career to embrace academic scholarship and who agreed to write the Afterword, and to my current Chair, Mack Ruffin, M.D, a consistently strong champion of scholarly work in Family Medicine.

Thank you also to Bill and Honey Jaffe, whose generous endowment has supported not only this book, but many other scholarly projects at the University Park (UP) Campus. I would like to recognize Pennsylvania Senator Jake Corman, as well, for his consistent support of the UP Campus, which has contributed significantly to its success and impacted positively on our region. In addition, our local hospital, Mount Nittany Medical Center, and each of the dedicated teaching physicians at our UP Campus deserve appreciation for their ongoing contribution to our students' medical education.

This list would not be complete without also acknowledging the staff at Atlantic Publishing for your artistic creativity and insightful guidance in bringing this project to fruition. I have learned much!

For their unfailing patience, understanding and support throughout my career and especially during this book project, I want to thank my wife, Cyndi, and our two children, Coral and Drew. I love you all.

Lastly, I want to thank the students at the Penn State College of Medicine UP Campus for being a consistent source of "positive deposits in my energy account". And finally, appreciation for choosing this book is extended to you, the reader, who is likely either cultivating in your own RMC garden, or perhaps contemplating planting the first seed.

Table of Contents

SECTION 3: IMAGES FROM REGIONAL MEDICAL CAMPUSES IN THE U.S. AND CANADA*

Author's Note

In the summer of 2014, I was asked to step into the role of interim Associate Dean for Education at the Penn State College of Medicine, University Park Campus. Although I had served as both a medical director and Vice-Chair for Family and Community Medicine at this campus for several years, I soon realized I had very little insight into all that is required to further develop and operate a regional medical campus (RMC). Nevertheless, I was confident that I could find and absorb the resources and knowledge necessary to serve in this role successfully, until we recruited a permanent new dean within the year. As a medical educator, this was something we had been teaching our medical students for years: identifying the appropriate resources and understanding how to seek out new knowledge through self-directed learning allows us to master the challenges that come with the rapidly developing field of medicine. As such, it was a rude awakening when I discovered that the resources available to guide those who are immersed in growing and operating a regional medical campus are significantly limited. I remember thinking how helpful it would have been to possess a guidebook for RMCs that I could refer to when needed. A book that provided insight into how other RMCs successfully operated, and one in which RMC champions shared their challenges and their solutions, would have been invaluable. At that time, such a resource did not exist.

By the following year, after we had recruited a new Associate Dean for Education and I had moved into the role of Assistant Dean for Student Affairs, I attended the Consortium of Longitudinal Integrated Clerkships (CLIC) annual conference in Asheville, North Carolina. As I was sitting with a group of colleagues in the small Asheville airport waiting to fly home, a fellow medical educator and friend, David Hirsch, M.D. (Harvard School of Medicine), shared how he and Ann Poncelet, M.D. (University of California-San Francisco School of Medicine) were working on a new book that would provide a guide to Longitudinal Integrated Clerkships (LIC). It was immediately clear how useful such a resource would be for those of us designing and delivering LICs at our own campuses, which were frequently regional campuses where innovative curricula were being piloted. On the flight home, I considered the idea of a similar guidebook for regional medical campuses that would share the experiences encountered and lessons learned by dedicated medical educators across the U.S. and Canada.

Subsequently, I discussed this book idea with leadership from the Group on Regional Medical Campuses (GRMC) of the Association of American Medical Colleges (AAMC) and received significant encouragement. Consequently, partnering with other Penn State colleagues, we delivered a presentation on the idea of developing a guidebook for RMCs at the 2016 Annual Spring GRMC Conference in Washington, D.C. The response was overwhelmingly positive, with multiple faculty members from numerous RMCs in the U.S. and Canada expressing their interest in participating as authors. Since then, it has been an ongoing collaboration between well over 50 contributing authors, the GRMC, AAMC representatives, my fellow Penn State faculty co-editors and our dedicated team at Atlantic Publishing. We designed the book to specifically encourage medical student co-authorship, since students at RMCs may, at times, have less opportunity for scholarship than their peers at major academic medical centers. We also made a decision that the primary motivation for this publication would be to share experiences and spread knowledge, as well as to promote scholarship and networking opportunities for RMC faculty and students. We decided from the beginning that no authors, from Penn State or elsewhere, would benefit financially from sales of the book. Instead, we would direct all author royalties into a fund to be used by the GRMC, with specific attention to supporting increased student involvement. In this way, since essentially all contributing authors were affiliated with the GRMC, everyone who contributed would benefit.

While this book is designed to provide immediate understanding and insight for those affiliated with current regional campuses, it is also a resource for those contemplating the development of future RMCs. In 2018, the AAMC released a report detailing a significant projected physician shortage in the U.S. by 2030.[1] This deficit is expected to affect all specialties and is directly related to the aging baby boomer population, who will require increasing healthcare, and the anticipated retirement of a significant proportion of currently practicing physicians. Approaches to meet this growing demand for more physicians include building new medical schools, expanding medical school class size at established academic medical centers, and creating regional medical campuses affiliated with established medical schools. Building completely new medical schools is cost-prohibitive for most communities. Many established medical schools have already expanded class size to accommodate more students, which stretches facility, research, and human resources to capacity. Alternatively, creating regional medical campuses at established medical facilities in a specific geographic area can create a cost-effective approach to increasing the number of physicians being trained. Consequently, both social and economic factors favor the continued development of RMCs. My hope is that this book will provide a valuable resource for all faculty, staff, and learners that find themselves looking toward regional medical campuses to train the next generation of physicians.

Michael P. Flanagan, M.D., FAAFP
Assistant Dean for Student Affairs
Professor and Vice-Chair of Family and Community Medicine
Penn State College of Medicine, University Park Campus

References:

1. Association of American Medical Colleges. 2018. *The Complexities of Physician Supply and Demand: Projections from 2016 to 2030. Final Report.*

Foreword

The statement, "If you've seen one regional campus, you've seen one regional campus", is one of the most common quotes heard at meetings of the Association of American Medical Colleges (AAMC) Group on Regional Medical Campuses (GRMC). Having spent 25 years of my professional career in a variety of roles at two regional campuses, I have experienced many opportunities and challenges associated with regional medical campuses. Even though I would prefer to focus on the opportunities, I think it is important that we also recognize many of the unique challenges related to regional campuses. As you will see, opportunities and challenges are frequently intertwined.

Some recognize the University of South Dakota, Sanford School of Medicine - Vermillion as the first U.S. regional medical campus (RMC). It was formed in 1907 as a two-year campus, but would not meet today's definition of a RMC. It became a four-year stand-alone medical school in 1977. The first regional campus by today's criteria[1] is the University of Tennessee Graduate School of Medicine in Knoxville, which was established in 1956 (AAMC data). There was a rapid growth of regional campuses in the 1970s, and again in the last decade, the latter driven primarily by a national call for increased medical school enrollment by 30 percent. According to the 2013-2016 AAMC Regional Medical Campus Survey, there are 115 regional medical campuses in the United States and Canada, 101 of which are in the U.S. The number of U.S.

medical schools with at least one regional campus is 48. Most regional campuses focus on third and fourth year clinical education. Another less common option is for a regional campus to focus on basic science education, typically in the first and/or second years[1]. In addition, there is a growing trend for regional campuses to provide the entire medical school experience, by providing all four (and sometimes three) years of medical education.

Regional campuses and other forms of community-based education continue to be a growing phenomenon across the U.S. and Canada. Dispersed education, especially in the clinical years, is becoming the rule rather than the exception, as the demands for quality clinical medical education increase. This is due to a variety of factors, including an increase in the number of medical students at most medical schools, the development of new medical schools, the increasing need for clinical sites to train other healthcare students, the increasing challenge of providing clinical education in large academic medical centers where providers are under increased expectations for clinical productivity, and the need to address specific mission areas such as rural, underserved, and primary care. Regional campuses often provide an environment where innovation in medical education can thrive. Recent workforce reports[2] demonstrate a need to increase medical school enrollment once again. As before, this is likely to result in an additional increase in the number (and importance) of regional medical campuses.

The Regional Medical Campus provides a rich mixture of topic-based chapters in Section 1, looking at a broad spectrum of opportunities and/ or challenges. Each author in this section has selected a topic that he or she felt qualified to address, based on their individual experience, and all chapters include both a faculty and medical student perspective. Section 2 provides an extensive sampling of different regional campuses across the United States and Canada. These campus descriptions provide a snapshot of 26 individual campuses, demonstrating their diversity, unique features, and commonalities.

The content of this book will be an invaluable resource to leaders who want to better understand the growing phenomenon of regional medical campuses, incorporate one or more regional campuses into their medical school, or make the most of the opportunities that already exist at their medical school. This book is not meant to provide a structured template, but instead will share examples of how other medical schools have incorporated regional campuses into their overall educational programs, and how they have engaged these campuses to meet unique needs or to address specific aspects of their overall mission.

E. Eugene Marsh, M.D.
Founding Senior Associate Dean
Professor of Neurology and Master Educator
Penn State College of Medicine, University Park Campus

References:

1. Cheifetz CE, McOwen KS, Gagne P, Wong JL. Regional Medical Campuses: A New Classification System. Academic Medicine 2014; 89:1140-1143.

2. Association of American Medical Colleges. 2018. *The Complexities of Physician Supply and Demand: Projections from 2016 to 2030. Final Report.*

SECTION 1

**Common Questions
and Solutions
Experienced At
Regional Medical
Campuses**

A — Developing a New Regional Medical Campus

1. Leading with Innovation

Authors:

- Ralitsa Akins, M.D., Ph.D.,
  Associate Dean of Faculty Affairs, Professor,
  Department of Medical Education and Clinical Sciences
  Washington State University, Elson S. Floyd College of Medicine

- Sahir "Sye" Jabbouri, MS I
  Washington State University,
  Elson S. Floyd College of Medicine, Everett Campus

Questions Addressed:

1. *How do you most effectively engage faculty to establish a new Regional Medical Campus?*

2. *How do you best engage students in experiencing a new regional campus for the first time?*

A Faculty Perspective:

Washington State University's Elson S. Floyd College of Medicine received accreditation in 2016. Starting a new medical school is a huge endeavor. Starting a medical school with the establishment of four clinical campuses could be even more challenging. The work with the clinical locations in Spokane, Everett, Vancouver, and Tri-cities started prior to receiving official accreditation; however, upon preliminary accreditation, the work accelerated, spanning from affiliation agreements to faculty recruitment to curriculum preparation on the clinical campuses. We were preparing to welcome 60 students and place 15 students on each of our four campuses as early as the third week of matriculation.

We planned and simultaneously implemented innovative programs for each of the clinical campuses:

(a) Expedited comprehensive and evidence-based faculty development

(b) Integrated curriculum with early clinical exposure, including six (6) week-long clinical experiences on campus, and

(c) Established a Community Hosting and Homestay Program, connecting medical students with families in their clinical campus community.

We approached faculty recruitment and faculty development simultaneously. Scheduling at least three on-site meetings at each campus, we reached out to the community physicians at times identified as convenient for them. For example, in Everett, we scheduled our visits for three hours on Saturday mornings, and provided breakfast for the attendees. It was critical to involve the leadership at the partnering institutions, who were the most enthusiastic supporters and did the "heavy lifting" of the sessions' advertisement to their physicians.

There are no guidelines on how to start faculty development programs in a new medical school. We decided to utilize an evidence-based perspective, starting with a literature review on faculty development, focusing on what other medical schools with clinical campuses have found effective, and identifying best practices and efficient tools. We reviewed the LCME publications on accreditation requirements and common deficiencies focused to faculty, especially as related to Standard 4. Another source of valuable information were discussions and presentations from the annual Learn Serve Lead AAMC meeting. We also reviewed our school's Strategic Plan and details in the Data Collection Instrument. Based on those findings, we designed a faculty development needs survey and disseminated it to current faculty as well as physicians from affiliated institutions on the four clinical campuses who had expressed a desire to join our faculty. Based on the needs survey, we designed a year-long schedule of faculty development sessions, with date, time, and location announced in advance, thus providing an opportunity for busy physicians to plan their schedules. A video-conference bridge was available for the vast majority of the sessions, allowing for remote participation and session recording. We presented a total of 73 sessions, reaching 303 individual physicians, and a total of 1,125 physician contacts. The number of attendees per session varied, based on topic and targeted audience. For example, small group sessions targeted course directors, and the large group sessions discussed curriculum, student evaluation, instructional methods, and scholarship.

It was important to provide a warm welcome to our affiliated institutions and the new faculty on all four campuses, express appreciation, and provide well-designed sessions with helpful information that they could use immediately during their first student encounter. We implemented a feedback reporting system, titled "You Said, We Did". After major sessions we emailed all participants additional information, answers to questions raised during the session, and a report on developments in which they were most interested.

The work at each campus was multifaceted, including completion of affiliation agreements, faculty recruitment, faculty development, and establishing a network for a student homestay program. This program allowed the students to stay with local families who introduced them to major local attractions and activities.

Student Perspective:

WSU College of Medicine's inaugural class began its medical school journey with the White Coat Ceremony, where speakers and attendees clearly declared their desire to support the students in excelling as future physicians. The clinical intersession week in Everett reinforced the deeply-felt support experienced during the White Coat Ceremony; physician preceptors, staff, and host families were genuinely invested in the success of the students. This strong sense of support bonded the students in their desire to give back to the Washington community.

The first week on the Everett campus began with students meeting their host families for the first time. Hosts included local physicians and other community members from various professions, all of whom were committed to serving the Everett community. The knowledge and experiences gained through this early participation in the Community Hosting and Homestay Program is critical, since these students will spend their last two years of medical school in Everett. Interactions with host families allowed students to learn about Everett and the challenges it faces, such as homelessness and drug abuse. During the Wednesday Community Night banquet, students networked with other host families and learned even more about the Everett community. The banquet also served as an opportunity for students to show appreciation to their host families, who opened their homes to them without hesitation.

Excitement was obvious among students as they toured the WSU Everett building, a four-story building which includes a café, a tiered lecture hall, numerous flat-screen TVs for video-conferencing, and several study areas to accommodate independent study as well as collaborative study. In addition, the engineering lab has high-quality technology including 3-D printers and scanners. The opportunities for innovation seemed limitless. For example, WSU medical students and engineering students could possibly collaborate to solve healthcare problems in Washington through technological innovation, thereby contributing to the Elson S. Floyd College of Medicine's mission statement.

During this intersession week, enthusiasm was also evident among faculty, staff, and guest speakers. It was no secret how excited they were to see the WSU College of Medicine's inaugural class in Everett, and they made sure the students knew it. A college of medicine dedicated to serving communities in Washington state builds high expectations, which is a mutual goal shared by all involved. Students engaged in a discussion on the importance of leadership in medicine and topics related to immunizations. They also gained hands-on experience administering subcutaneous and intramuscular injections with the guidance of Everett's Associate Dean of Clinical Education and a nurse from the community. Hands-on instruction with a ratio of one faculty to seven or eight students maximized the learning experience and gave students confidence in the knowledge and skills they gained to administer subcutaneous and intramuscular injections in real patients.

The most significant highlight of the clinical intersession was the actual clinical experience. For example, in just two days, a student worked in the emergency department, a family medicine clinic, and an outpatient orthopedic surgery clinic. In addition to being exposed to different medical fields, students learned from the physician preceptors the basics of clinical reasoning and interpreting clinical tests such as CT scans and lab reports. Preceptors also encouraged students to take an active role in patient care by taking a patient history and performing heart and lung auscultations.

Overall, the warm welcome, enthusiasm, support, and leadership that WSU medical students experienced during the first week on their clinical campus made them eager to return to the Everett community for their next clinical intersession. Having this clinical experience early on in medical school serves as a great reminder of the end goal and motivates students to thrive.

References:

1. Karen Leslie, M.D., MEd, Lindsay Baker, MEd, Eileen Egan-Lee, MEd, Martina Esdaile, MA, and Scott Reeves, PhD, MSc. (July, 2013). Advancing Faculty Development in Medical Education: A Systematic Review. Academic Medicine, 88(7): 1038-1045.

2. John P. Langlois, M.D., and Sarah B. Thach, MPH. (2003). Bringing Faculty Development to Community-based Preceptors. Academic Medicine 78(2): 150-155.

3. Michelle McLean, Francois Cilliers and Jacqueline M. Van Wyk. (2008). Faculty development: Yesterday, today and tomorrow. Medical Teacher, 30:555-584.

4. Scott E. Moser, M.D.; John N. Dorsch, MD; Rick Kellerman, MD. (2004). The RAFT Approach to Academic Detailing with Preceptors. Fam Med 36(5):316-8.

5. Yvonne Steinert, Mary Ellen Macdonald, Miriam Boillat, Michelle Elizov, Sarkis Meterissian, Saleem Razack, Marie-Noel Ouellet,and Peter J McLeod. (2010). Faculty development: if you build it, they will come. Medical Education, 44: 900-907.

Summary points:

- Starting a new medical school with multiple clinical campuses requires attention to both the big picture (recruiting faculty, affiliation agreements, etc.), and to the details (faculty development, instructional methodology, assessment and scholarship, wellness, and building meaningful interpersonal relationships).

- Early exposure to the clinical campus and utilization of a homestay program for students to connect with local families eases student integration in the new environment and helps them feel at home.

- The warm welcome and enthusiasm that the medical students experience during the first week on their campus make them eager to return to the community for their next clinical experience.

2. Medical Student Influence on Solving Challenges Associated with Creating a New Regional Medical Campus

Authors:

- Pierre Gagné, M.D., FRCP(C), MSc.
  Senior Advisor for Regional Medical Campus Development;
  Professor of Nuclear Medicine, *Campus de l'UdeM en Mauricie,
  Faculté de médecine, Université de Montréal.*

- Patrice Levasseur-Fortin MS II,
  President, Medical Student Association- RMC Chapter,
  *Campus de l'UdeM en Mauricie, Faculté de médecine,
  Université de Montréal.*

- Pierre-Luc Dazé M.D. Clinical Faculty, Emergency Medicine,
  *Campus de l'UdeM en Mauricie, Faculté de médecine,
  Université de Montréal.*

Questions Addressed:

1. *What are the main challenges related to the development of a new RMC and what strategies could be useful to overcome those challenges relative to the students' perspective?*

2. *How can faculty and students join forces in creating a new RMC and how might this look?*

A Faculty Perspective:

The physician shortage was so severe in the Mauricie region of Quebec in 2003 that it mandated an urgent solution to enhance the attraction and retention of new physicians in the area. Recognizing that providing medical education to students locally would be an efficient strategy to achieve this[1], the Mauricie RMC was started within a period of 14 months. This extended from the meeting of the Faculté de Médecine de l'Université de Montréal (UdeM) and Mauricie's regional hospital, the Centre Hospitalier Régional de Trois-Rivières (CHRTR), to the admission of the first cohort into the pre-medical year in 2004. Thirty students were admitted into the first medical year in 2005, and the cycle continued to include the full M.D. program (pre-med year + 4 M.D. years). This fast track was made possible by implementing a copy-paste formula where the same program was given at the same time to all medical students at both the Montreal and Mauricie campuses. Even though this strategy minimized the complexity of starting a regional campus, many challenges appeared.

Medical teaching building (MTB):

Starting so fast had a negative drawback: the loss of negotiating power with the unique funding agent, the provincial government. Hence, the MTB was inaugurated after significant political challenges and delays in 2009. The local university, the Université du Québec à Trois-Rivières, which already hosted and provided the pre-medical year, became the foster home for medical students from 2004 until 2009. The Université de Montréal's (UdeM) presence was eclipsed by the Université du Québec à Trois-Rivières (UQTR), and some medical students even started to identify themselves as UQTR Medical School students to the dismay of the UdeM authorities.

Expect the unexpected:

Although every IT expert provided assurances that video-conferences between Montreal and the Mauricie region would cause no problems, we soon found out that we had to have a Plan B and often a Plan C. Connectivity issues were caused, among other factors, by the presence of a bridge to link the two different IT pipelines involved in medical education, one for healthcare and a second for education. Unexpected failures occurred, and an IT specialist had to be on call for real-time interventions at each site for any video-conference session.

Taming the Tiger:

The class size was very large in Montreal, with 260 first-year medical students attending a formal lecture in a single auditorium. All the initial lectures were given by the main campus teachers in the Montreal campus classrooms. Most often questions by the audience were not heard by the regional campus audience of 30 first-year students, which increased medical student anxiety. When students asked questions, the camera zoomed in on their face, which appeared on the large screen at the central campus! This decreased their willingness to ask questions. When the video-conference link was completely lost for many minutes, the class had to be interrupted on both campuses until a recording of each video-conference was operational. We found the best solution was to reverse the process and bring the teachers from Montreal to the regional campus and send the lecture back through video-conference to the Montreal-based students. Once the faculty had been at the regional campus, they simply fell in love with its medical students and staff. This had a therapeutic effect on both the students and faculty, but had to be repeated often, as the UdeM faculty is quite large.

Another useful strategy was to intermingle regional campus faculty into the numerous medical program committees, at all possible levels. Again, getting to know each other created emotional bonds and alleviated the "us versus them" attitude.

A problem-solving committee (PSC) was created with the creation of the regional campus. Medical student representatives sat on this committee and were responsible for bringing back identified problems to the regional campus for review. The PSC was presided over by the Regional Dean, and several medical education directors from the regional and central campuses sat on this committee, including the program director, clerkship directors, and a small group of clinical teaching representatives. Through their PSC representatives, medical students from the regional campus were able to express their frustrations without restrictions. The PSC kept track of student complaints, identifying who was responsible for addressing them and the timeline associated with solutions.

A Student Perspective:

The delays in building the Medical Teaching Building did not decrease student anxiety or the feeling of serving as guinea pigs. As we spent most of our time at the Université du Québec à Trois-Rivières (UQTR), we came to embrace its culture. We began to attend joint social events with other healthcare student associations at the UQTR, such as Podiatrics. Concurrently, we had excellent support and communication with the l'Université de Montréal medical student association in Montreal. As such, we became hybrid students and felt empowered as each aspect of the regional campus had to be created. Knowing the Mauricie population supported the construction of the Medical Teaching Building through a philanthropic $1 million donation, we found numerous ways to give back to the Mauricie community. For example, we participated in a mega-marathon between the Montreal and Mauricie campuses through an annual fundraising event where teams of medical students are sponsored to run 100 miles from Montreal to the Mauricie campuses, in multiple 5K relays. We actively participated in the design of the Medical Teaching Building through every step from beginning to completion. It is now the heart of our Mauricie Regional Medical Campus. As a smaller campus, we felt we had excellent internal communication within our campus. For example, if we needed to address an urgent issue, the medical student representatives could go from class to class and receive direct feedback from all regional campus medical students.

Video-conferencing was a tough challenge. This evolved to the point where we did not feel comfortable asking questions. The fear of having a sub-par medical education was solved by the publication of comparative scores between the two campuses at critical points in the curriculum. We also feared that being away from the main campus could jeopardize our ability to pursue a competitive residency, such as Pediatrics. The match results proved we had the same opportunities with no fewer challenges, but an equal chance for success.

We fully participated in the Problem Solving Committee. We had a major issue when intercampus transfers were initially denied. This resulted in a serious accreditation citation. From that moment, we learned to put aside our personal opinions and to speak on behalf of the whole medical student population. We also made sure every voice was heard and did not underreport potential issues.

Currently, we feel privileged to have an excellent relationship with the Mauricie Regional Campus Dean, as well as its faculty and staff. We created numerous philanthropic and social initiatives to give back to the population in return for the opportunity to receive our medical education in such an environment. Indeed, serving our community has become a core value for our campus.

References:

1. Brooks, Robert G. M.D.; Walsh, Michael; Mardon, Russell E. Ph.D.; Lewis, Marie MPH; Clawson, Art M.S. The Roles of Nature and Nurture in the Recruitment and Retention of Primary Care Physicians in Rural Areas: A Review of the Literature. Acad Med. 2002 Aug;77(8):790-8

Summary points:

- **Adaptability.** Expect the unexpected, as numerous challenges will occur at both the student and institutional levels.

- **Communication.** Students must be able to address issues in a structured approach with the appropriate authorities.

- **Representation.** Opinions expressed by student representatives should reflect the majority's position, not their own.

- **Challenges.** Intercampus transfer, video-conference connectivity, regional campus students' fear of being perceived as second-class citizens, and the creation of a student hybrid identity were challenging issues we encountered.

- **Community.** A smaller-scale campus enhances the student's sense of belonging and empowerment.

B Admissions, Orientation, and Recruitment

1. How to Develop a Student-Engaged Admissions Process at a Regional Medical Campus

Authors:

- Morgan Decker MS I,
  Penn State College of Medicine, University Park Campus

- Melissa Vayda, Ed.D., Director, Educational Affairs,
  Penn State College of Medicine, University Park Campus

- Jeffrey G. Wong, M.D., Associate Dean for Medical Education,
  Penn State College of Medicine, University Park Campus

Questions Addressed:

1. *How can medical students become involved in the admissions process at a Regional Medical Campus (RMC)?*

2. *How does a RMC interface with the admissions process at the main campus?*

A Faculty Perspective:

Background:

While medical student participation in admissions is common at most medical schools, the extent to which Regional Medical Campus (RMC) students participate in the process is highly variable. In 2016, the Penn State College of Medicine (PSCOM) began work on establishing a four-year curriculum of study using a newly designed innovative program at the University Park (UP) Regional Medical Campus. We describe the details of our students' involvement in admissions, which serve as a model for other RMCs that wish to significantly incorporate students into the admissions process.

Admissions:

As we developed the Admissions Program for the RMC, the initial stages of the process remained at the main campus in Hershey. Medical student aspirants applied, were interviewed, and were ultimately accepted to the PSCOM through the same selection criteria and process as all applicants. As part of the secondary American Medical Colleges Application Service (AMCAS) application to PSCOM, applicants had the opportunity to express interest in specialized programs or locations, including being considered for assignment to the new track at the University Park RMC. Once accepted into PSCOM, those applicants who expressed interest in attending the RMC were identified and a site-selection process was begun.

Expressed Interest:

The RMC Student Services office developed profiles on each student applicant who expressed interest in the regional campus. Prospective applicants were personally contacted by the medical students on the RMC admissions team, to verify interest and to provide additional information on the site-selection process. Through the substance of these individual conversations, student applicants either chose to disengage or expressed continued interest in the process. Supplemental mailings from the Student Services office provided additional details about the new program.

The medical student representatives interacted frequently with potential applicants, and by design, were given a significant level of autonomy when interacting with candidates. Through this iterative communication process, the medical students on the site-selection team were able to determine which candidates were should be invited to participate in a "UP Preview" event which was a requirement for further consideration of assignment to the University Park RMC.

University Park Site-Selection Process:

A UP Preview event was developed to help screen candidates and select for specific characteristics deemed to fit with our new curriculum. Sensitivity to group dynamics, working within a peer-learning team, being self-directed in one's learning, and general comfort with creating, rather than following structure, were felt to be essential qualities for predicting success in our innovative curriculum. In contradistinction to many traditional medical school interview days, the UP Preview event engaged student applicants in a series of group problem-solving activities, as well as six Multiple Mini-Interview-like "dialogues" that were subsequently evaluated by the interviewers themselves.

All students were observed and evaluated by each member of the RMC admissions team, comprised of medical student representatives, faculty, staff, and a patient who lives in the local community. Each member submitted an evaluation for each participant. A simple three-point scale was used to rank the following categories for each applicant: enthusiasm, communication, self-awareness, social confidence, curiosity, ability to connect ideas, perseverance, and genuine interest in the program.

Once the evaluation data were tallied and the final ranking process performed, those applicants rated at the top of the list were offered assignment to the University Park RMC program. If they declined, they still remained enrolled in the main campus program. A "waiting-list" for initially less highly ranked applicants was used to subsequently fill the available positions at the RMC. It was evident that our choice to deeply involve medical students in the site-selection process at our RMC proved to be both highly valuable and effective.

A Student Perspective:

The Process:

As a medical student representative for the Admissions Committee, my responsibilities began when I received a list of interested candidates. A personalized, introductory email was sent to those individuals, including my contact information and a conferencing request to both answer questions and assess interest. A common communication method that suited both parties was video-conferencing. Phone calls were also utilized. From that pool, I selected candidates who demonstrated genuine interest in our program and extended them an invitation to the UP Preview event, which was comprised of informational sessions, interviews, group activities, and social functions. All of the information gathered during this process was utilized by our team to determine acceptances.

Reflections:

While many medical schools incorporate students in their admissions activities, the amount of responsibility associated with the process outlined above far surpasses intermittent participation. Until the campus event, I had primary responsibility for communicating with, assessing, and offering an interview invitation to my assigned candidates. It was a very consuming process due to the significant time commitment, but the dedicated effort proved to be vital. We were able to select a class that is unique, engaged, and, most importantly, cohesive. Their group dynamics not only facilitate learning, but contribute to our culture of teamwork. As a student, assuming a significant portion of the admissions process was especially rewarding.

The Big Picture:

Tailoring the admissions process to your campus and its philosophies is critical for selecting the appropriate candidates. As a RMC, we took advantage of our applicant pool size to effectively screen candidates at the deepest level. Five medical students were on the RMC site-selection team, and we were each assigned approximately 20 students. Individually, we spent about three hours speaking with each of our assigned candidates. Our team decided to establish and maintain an open line of communication during the entire process to ensure that we developed meaningful relationships. In addition, we agreed to promote a culture of transparency, tackling the hard questions with straightforward, honest answers while simultaneously recognizing that ours was not the program for all candidates and vice versa. Being honest with our applicants, but also with ourselves, helped to resolve any anxieties from both parties. While our process required additional time, we felt it was extremely effective for selecting the appropriate candidates.

Summary points:

- RMCs, by the nature of their curricula, may have important and unique considerations for applicants that differ from students matriculating at the main campus.

- Because of these unique considerations, traditional medical school interview days may not be the most effective process for selecting applicants.

- Medical students can be valuable and effective participants in the admissions selection process. The smaller and more intimate size of a RMC should be used to the benefit of the existing medical students on the admissions team in helping to select their future colleagues.

2. Student Selection of a Regional Medical Campus

Authors:

- Michael Robinson, Ph.D.,
  Associate Dean for Foundational Sciences,
  University of Kansas School of Medicine–Salina

- Luke Johnson MS III,
  University of Kansas School of Medicine–Salina

Questions Addressed:

1. *Why do students choose to study at a Regional Medical Campus rather than the main campus?*

2. *How does the Regional Medical Campus attract and select their students for their campus?*

A Faculty Perspective:

The rural Regional Medical Campus (RMC) of the University of Kansas School of Medicine (KUSM) in Salina, Kansas (KUSM-Salina) originated from the need to train physicians who would serve rural Kansas. Established in 2011 with an annual matriculation of eight students, KUSM-Salina was accredited as a four-year campus by the LCME, employing an identical curriculum to the main Kansas City campus[1]. Salina is in a predominantly agricultural area 180 miles west of Kansas City in central Kansas. With a small class size, attracting the most suitable candidates is crucial. Rural applicants constitute the majority of students who select the Salina campus. Often, these applicants have different experiences than students from urban areas and, as a consequence, may not appear as competitive to the selection committee. All KUSM-Salina applicants are processed and selected through a central committee of the KUSM.

Inspiring rural students to consider a career in medicine can be challenging. Shadowing experiences are more difficult in rural areas making it difficult for applicants to obtain meaningful medical experience. To address this, KUSM has established a pipeline initiative called the Scholars in Rural Health Program. Offered during the final two undergraduate years, the program provides guaranteed medical school admission to successful rural applicants provided they maintain required academic and professional standards. Interestingly, many students accepted into the program have chosen to matriculate at the Kansas City or Wichita campuses rather than returning to the rural Salina campus. To date, students appear more likely to migrate to Kansas City from rural Kansas than the reverse. Nevertheless, an inspiring core of students have been attracted to Salina by the smaller community, smaller numbers of faculty, more intimate atmosphere, less competition for study space, and a closer relationship to both teaching faculty and administration.

Additional challenges that the Salina campus faces include the lower availability of laboratory research opportunities, and lack of free-clinic experiences (contrasted with the JayDoc clinics available in both Kansas City and Wichita). Thus, to better compete for quality students, KUSM-Salina does offer:

1.   Generous scholarships from local and regional benefactors,

2. Outstanding clinical teaching and hands-on experiences with enthusiastic clinical faculty, and

3. An interactive faculty/administration environment that is able to respond quickly and efficiently to administrative and academic problems.

To this point, the biggest marketing asset of our program has been our students who work tirelessly as enthusiastic ambassadors for the Salina campus.

A Student Perspective:

The Salina campus of the University of Kansas School of Medicine is one of two KUSM Regional Medical Campuses (RMCs). Students who are invited to interview are generally offered their choice of campus. The particular advantages of the Salina campus include:

1. An accessible administration,
2. A 1:1 physician-student ratio, and
3. Early exposure to active roles in patient care.

These qualities, combined with a mission to serve underserved and rural populations, are generally the most common reasons students choose to attend KUMC-Salina.

An important part of any medical school is its administration. The KUMC-Salina administration is a particular strength. Administrative personnel are always readily available to discuss student concerns and have demonstrated a willingness to implement policy change in a prompt manner when appropriate. Students often present questions, concerns, and/or requests to the administration and receive a response within a week. This prompt attention to detail increases student satisfaction and serves as a living example of continuous process improvement for students and faculty alike.

The KUMC-Salina clinical opportunities are one of the greatest strengths of the campus. A 1:1 physician to student ratio provides excellent clinical teaching, particularly with regard to:

1. Patient presentation skills
2. Clinical care (significant responsibilities on clinical rounds)
3. A significant role for inpatient admissions

In addition, it is common for first- and second-year medical students at KUMC-Salina to be first assist on deliveries and surgeries. These experiences continue into the third and fourth years, in which students are given even larger patient care roles as they prepare for residency.

There are several downsides to the KUMC-Salina campus that are important to recognize. The small class size can result in conflict between individuals, which may be difficult to resolve. Also, most lectures are delivered by professors in Kansas City making complex queries problematic.

To date, the performance of KUMC-Salina students on standardized high-stakes exams has been equivalent to their counterparts on other campuses. Students studying in Salina feel that they are exceptionally well-prepared for their residencies by attending a RMC.

References:

1. Cathcart-Rake W, Robinson M, Paolo A. From Infancy to Adolescence: The Kansas University School of Medicine-Salina: A Rural Medical Campus Story. Academic Medicine. 2016;92(5):622-7.

Summary points:

- The University of Kansas School of Medicine at Salina is the smallest allopathic medical school campus in the country with an annual intake of eight students.

- Most KUMC-Salina students are from a rural background and wish to practice in a rural setting.

- Attracting qualified students to Salina is a major focus.

- Students coming to Salina are attracted by scholarship support, familiarity with administration and an excellent clinical experience.

- The downsides of the Salina campus include distance from main campus teaching faculty and resolving potential friction between students.

Medical Education and Curriculum Development

1. Adopting Orphan Topics into the Clinical Curriculum

Authors:

- Brook A. Hubner, M.Ed.,
  Director of Medical Student Affairs,
  University of Alabama (UAB) School of Medicine,
  Tuscaloosa Regional Campus

- Danielle Fincher, MS IV,
  University of Alabama School of Medicine,
  Tuscaloosa Regional Campus

- Mary Craig, MS III,
  University of Alabama School of Medicine,
  Tuscaloosa Regional Campus

- Mary Katherine Sweeney, MS III,
  University of Alabama School of Medicine,
  Tuscaloosa Regional Campus

Questions Addressed:

1. *How might academic medical school faculty create a curriculum that develops a culture of inclusion, fosters professional growth and development, and supports student success?*

2. *What do medical students perceive to be important aspects of this type of curriculum?*

A Faculty Perspective:

The rapidly changing health care landscape requires physicians to have more than book knowledge, procedural skills, and critical thinking ability. The Liaison Committee on Medical Education and the Carnegie Foundation's 2010 report call for cultural competence and the "progressive formation of the physician's professional identity" as an integral part of medical education reform.

It is incumbent on medical educators to tap into students' capacity for conceptual creativity, tolerance for ambiguity, and personal insight in ways that move beyond traditional clinical education. Medical educators do this, in part, by raising students' social and cultural awareness and encouraging them to critically evaluate the multifaceted health care issues they face as students and will continue to face as practicing physicians. On the UAB School of Medicine's Tuscaloosa Regional Campus, we tackled this by developing a curriculum of "orphan" topics not part of traditional medical education, but important to professional development.

Creating an orphan topic curriculum:

To provide an environment conducive to culturally-inclusive, patient-centered professional development in third and fourth year medical students, the Dean, Student Affairs Director, and students developed these orphan topics into a year-long, "Dean's Hour" curriculum.

The Dean's role as an active participant allows him to role model reflection, constructive discourse, and critical inquiry. Just as importantly, the time allows students to interact informally with the Dean, student affairs leadership, and each other. The sessions foster the development of a community of learners and provide mentoring and encouragement to reflect on and make sense of life experiences. We initially carved out one hour, twice a month at noon from the clerkship schedule, operating under the notion that if we feed them they will come. Over time, Dean's Hour has evolved to include a new School of Medicine learning community curriculum and is now a weekly event.

Structure and Content:

The schedule design was driven by the regional campus Dean's availability, given his desire to facilitate sessions and know the students personally. Third-year students have this time blocked in their clerkship schedules; fourth-year students come when their schedules permit and provide valuable peer mentoring, support, and a more experienced voice to the discussions. Providing a lunchtime discussion format and restricting attendance to students, invited guests, Student Affairs Director, and Dean creates a relaxed, protected space for students to converse and reflect. We purposely include topics that will challenge students to examine their preconceived notions and explore other points of view.

Broadly, Dean's Hour topics fall into three categories: culture of inclusion, professional roles and development, and student success. Our discussants include everyone from the mayor to hospital chaplain, faculty, and community members. We invite speakers to share their knowledge with the students, but ask that they limit PowerPoint slides and instead engage the students in conversations about the topic.

Selected Topics

Culture of Inclusion	Physician Leadership; Professional Roles	Student Success
Caring for the disabled patient	Conflict of Interest: Perspectives from research, pharmacy, and medicine	Career planning
Challenging patients: understanding why patients don't/won't/can't comply	Health Care Leadership / Hospital Systems: a hospital CEO's perspective	Professionalism: reporting a concern
LGBTQAI+ patient populations	Social responsibility and engaging a community	Stress management
Referring patients for social services: what happens after the referral?	Impaired physicians: warning signs, resources, interventions	Success on your clerkships
Spirituality & Medicine	Intersection of medicine and the law: legal issues, malpractice, regulatory compliance	Finding work/life balance

Topics are scheduled to align with the natural rhythms of third year. Initially, we provide big idea topics and sessions that will help the student make the transition from pre-clinical to clinical education. Later, we present topics that complement patient interactions. At the end of the year, sessions allow for synthesis and evaluation of clinical experiences. By this point, students are comfortable asking hard questions and challenging pre-conceived notions as a fully-developed community of learners. Feedback from the students indicate these sessions are well-received and an important part of the clinical learning experience.

Student Perspectives:

A successful physician studies the art of medicine beyond the closed doors of the hospital and has extended her knowledge base to include topics related to, but too often deemed nonessential to, clinical care. Creating a curriculum and learning environment that fosters professional growth during the clinical years is a unique way to expand learning to topics that may not be taught elsewhere, but that are important to integrate with the clinical curriculum.

Students appreciate topics that foster personal and professional development and this is the perfect place for us to begin to develop tools that we can use while in school and throughout our professional lives. We found it helpful that some Dean's Hours incorporated topics that we can practice in a safe space, then immediately use on our clinical rotations or in our daily lives.

Early in the year, a clinical psychologist led us in a chocolate tasting mindfulness practice so that we could learn to practice mindfulness and learn about the impact mindfulness can have on our role as physicians. It was an interactive, enjoyable way to introduce students to a mindfulness practice. Later in the year, a session with the hospital chaplain challenged us to think about how we view death, how we think our patients view death, and what a transition from hospital to hospice can do for patients and families. The next week some of us used these skills when discussing a patient in our service and the value of a chaplain consult.

Focusing on specific areas of student interest helps us stay engaged and fosters self-directed learning. We are encouraged to suggest ideas or topics. By following through with those suggestions, the administration conveys an important message that they care about each of us as students and support our individual interests and passions. In addition, supplementing discussions with relevant articles from academic sources and popular media encourages us to contribute to curriculum development and provides opportunities for additional exploration.

We appreciate having protected time to come together informally in a safe space. A relaxed, conversational format allows us to use a different part of our brains, and group discussions, activities, and reflections are refreshingly different from a traditional lecture format. We appreciate that most topics are directly applicable to medicine and patient interactions, but are delivered in a way that moves beyond clinical learning. Discussions during lunch on Friday afternoons are an effective way to broaden our scope of knowledge, better prepare us for our future professional roles, and build relationships that foster a sense of community.

References:

1. Association of American Medical Colleges. (2005). Cultural Competence Education [Brochure]. Author. Retrieved November 18, 2016, from https://www.aamc.org/download/54338/data/culturalcomped.pdf.

2. Hirsh, D. A., Ogur, B., Thibault, G. E., & Cox, M. (2007). "Continuity" as an organizing principle for clinical education reform. *New England Journal of Medicine*, 356(8), 858.

3. Irby, D. M., Cooke, M., & O'Brien, B. C. (2010). Calls for reform of medical education by the Carnegie Foundation for the Advancement of Teaching: 1910 and 2010. *Academic Medicine*, 85(2), 220-227.

Summary points:

- Medical educators should raise students' social and cultural awareness, encourage them to become comfortable with ambiguity, and develop their capacity for reflection and insight beyond traditional clinical education.

- An "orphan topic" curriculum can help develop a culture of inclusion, foster professional growth and development, and support student success.

- Developing a progression of topics that align with the natural rhythms of third year helps build meaning and value.

- Encouraging student input in curriculum development increases engagement and satisfaction and fosters self-directed learning.

- Providing a safe, restricted meeting space helps develop a community of learners and provides mentoring and encouragement to reflect on and make sense of life experiences.

- Creating a curriculum that encourages patient centeredness, social awareness, flexibility, resilience, and leadership promotes medical student professional development and provides essential tools for student success.

2. Peer-Led Didactics

Authors:

- Christine Waasdorp Hurtado, M.D., MSCS, FAAP,
  Director for Didactics and Longitudinal Curriculum,
  Associate Professor of Pediatrics,
  University of Colorado School of Medicine
  Colorado Springs Branch

- Jacob Fox MS III,
  University of Colorado School of Medicine
  Colorado Springs Branch

- Chad L. Stickrath, M.D., FACP,
  Assistant Dean for Education,
  Associate Professor of Medicine,
  University of Colorado School of Medicine
  Colorado Springs Branch

Questions Addressed:

1. *Should students lead didactic sessions for their peer group?*

2. *What training is needed for students and faculty to facilitate such student-led sessions?*

3. *How can students and faculty maximize the effectiveness of these peer group sessions?*

A Faculty Perspective:

Why peer-led didactics?

Student-led didactics can be effectively utilized to cover curricular content during clinical years. The benefits of this methodology likely outweigh the risks, or burdens. Peer teaching has been shown to improve knowledge outcomes and durability of learning in peer teachers.[1] In addition, the peer-teaching model produces non-inferior[2], or possibly superior, outcomes in peer learners compared to a faculty-taught model. Peer learners have shown a preference for peer teaching which may reflect the level of interaction, pace of the lecture, appropriateness of the material, and comfort within the environment.[3] Finally, since residents must be prepared to teach and evaluate medical students, peer teaching experiences as medical students may improve future teaching skills necessary during residency training.

How should peer-led didactics be developed and organized? Determining Goals and Objectives:

Prior to developing objectives for each peer-led clinical session, faculty must coordinate with main campus core clinical specialty directors and curriculum leaders to ensure comparability of goals and objectives. In our curriculum, we utilized the university curriculum map and learning objectives from the main campus clinical blocks to develop our teaching plan.

Creating the Lesson Plan:

Several strategies can improve the efficacy of the didactic curriculum, including: incorporating active learning concepts (e.g. flipped-classroom concepts, case-based learning), utilizing frequent retrieval practice (e.g. frequent low-stakes quizzes), spacing learning of concepts over time, and interweaving different types of content throughout the curriculum.[4] Just as faculty educational experts guide the organization of the curriculum as a whole, faculty content experts should closely guide the development of individual sessions.

For our curriculum, which was based on a Longitudinal Integrated Clerkship (LIC) model and covered objectives from all ten core clinical specialties, we blocked one afternoon (two to four hours) per week for didactics. Didactic sessions were scheduled according to the developmental needs of the students, with specialty and other types of content intermixed. Specialty topics related to NBME subject exams were covered a few weeks prior to that upcoming subject exam.

At the beginning of the academic year, students received a list of topics to be covered throughout the year and they selected one or two topics to teach during the year. Seven weeks prior to an assigned session, students received the required learning objectives and faculty-mentor assignment. Over a four to six week time frame, students developed the session with their assigned faculty member with oversight by educational leaders. Each student-faculty team created an interactive presentation that included case-based material. They utilized a combination of slideshow, case- and problem-based learning, algorithm development, and games (e.g. game-show formats). Pre-reading was identified and delivered to students prior to each session. Students led the didactic session while faculty provided support through personal examples and insights, answering questions, and ensuring the accuracy of the materials and discussion.

Orientation and Education for Students and Faculty:

Faculty and students should receive education on high-yield teaching strategies. Mayer's principles for effective PowerPoint should be reviewed, including: simple backgrounds, limited text, highlighting critical information, consideration of spatial contiguity, and purposeful use of images.[5] It may be beneficial to educate students on how to effectively facilitate discussions, elicit audience engagement, and answer questions in an engaging manner. Education on giving and receiving feedback on educational sessions will ultimately improve outcomes and satisfaction.

Evaluation, Lessons Learned, and Next Steps:

Our first class rated peer-led didactics second only to self-study as their most valuable learning modality, while faculty-led didactics were met with mixed reviews. Students met or exceeded the national average on all NBME shelf exams.

Didactics should be scheduled to minimize disruption to student clinical schedules and should be brief to optimize attention and participation. Formative feedback to student-teachers and faculty should be provided after every session to improve teaching effectiveness. Subsequently, we increased the number of didactic sessions each student leads and have created a menu of teaching strategies to assist in session planning. Learning objectives are shared with the entire class a week before each session to guide independent study. A teaching boot camp for students during orientation at the beginning of the year is provided to increase teaching effectiveness, and similar concepts are emphasized during faculty development sessions.

A Student Perspective:

What are the components of effective peer-led didactics?

In the clinical years, students are expected to employ independent learning. A successful student must be engaged, proactive, self-motivated, and willing to seek out learning opportunities. We believe that effective peer-led didactics should be tailored for the learner's increasing responsibility and independence. Student-teachers may make learning material available before the session in the form of worksheets, algorithms, practice questions, pre-recorded lectures uploaded to YouTube, or other web-based modalities to allow students to engage the material at their convenience. In their lessons, peer-educators should emphasize "high-yield" material — concepts relevant to clinical clerkships, NMBE exams, and patient care — and avoid recapitulating knowledge from pre-clinical years. Peer-led didactics should mirror patient-centered learning that occurs on the wards and lessons should be problem- or case-based to engage fellow students.

What are the potential benefits of peer-led didactics?

Effective peer-led didactics benefit both learners and the peer-teacher. The audience's familiarity with fellow peer-teachers may enhance attention and help foster a comfortable learning environment in which students feel less afraid to participate. Moreover, since peer-teachers have an understanding of current student pre-clinical and clinical knowledge, they can tailor material to an appropriate level of understanding and connect with fellow students on a more personal level. Peer-led didactics enables students to practice the educator role, which students will seek to refine and master through residency and beyond. This model provides a learning opportunity for peer-teachers to choose a subject, to evaluate primary and secondary literature resources during construction of the lesson and to become an "expert" in the delivery of that content. Finally, weekly class meetings confer a social benefit as students enjoy the opportunity to support one another.

What are the Challenges of peer-led didactics?

The primary challenge to peer-led didactics is suboptimal teaching and delivery of content. Peer-teachers who do not prepare well for their session often default to ineffective teaching practices including lectures without audience engagement, repetition of pre-clinical material without clinical or NBME exam correlates, inappropriate scope of lessons, and ineffective visual aids such as text-dense slides. To help protect against suboptimal teaching, students should work closely with their faculty-mentor to ensure a focus on "high-yield" material. Remedies for poor teaching include immediate post-session feedback, improved education on how to teach at the beginning of the year, allowing peer-teachers to lead lessons that interest them, and encouragement from the faculty towards innovation and creativity in the lesson design.

References:

1. Gregory A, Walker I, McLaughlin K, Peets AD. (2011). Both preparing to teach and teaching positively impact learning outcomes for peer teachers. Med Teach, 33, e417-22

2. Rudland JR, Rennie SC. (2014). Medical faculty opinions of peer tutoring. Educ for Health, 7:4-9

3. Jayakumar N, Srirathan D, Shah R, Jakubowska A, Clarke A, Annan D, et al. (2016). Which peer teaching methods do medical students prefer? Educ Health, 29, 142-7

4. Brown PC, Roediger HL, McDaniel MA. (2014). Make it Stick. The Science of Successful Learning. Cambridge, MA. Belknap Press.

5. Mayer, RE. (2010). Applying the science of learning to medical education. Medical Education, 44, 543–549.

Summary points:

- Peer-teaching has been shown to improve knowledge outcomes and durability of learning in peer-teachers.

- Peer-teaching experiences as medical students may improve future teaching skills necessary during residency training.

- Faculty and students should receive education on high-yield teaching strategies

- A teaching boot camp for students during orientation at the beginning of the year can be provided to increase student teaching effectiveness.

- To help protect against suboptimal teaching, students should work closely with their faculty-mentor to ensure a focus on "high-yield" material.

3. Creating a Nutrition Curriculum

Authors:

- Adrienne N. Zavala, M.D.,
  Assistant Professor of Family Medicine,
  West Virginia University School of Medicine,
  Eastern Campus

- Rosemarie Cannarella Lorenzetti M.D., MPH,
  Associate Dean of Student Services,
  Professor of Family Medicine,
  West Virginia University School of Medicine,
  Eastern Campus

- Alaina Thiel MS IV;
  West Virginia University School of Medicine,
  Eastern Campus

Questions Addressed:

1. *What practical nutritional information is most important for students to share with patients during their third year, and how can this be incorporated into the curriculum?*

2. *How do we tech Motivational Interviewing as part of our Nutrition curriculum?*

A Faculty Perspective:

It is widely acknowledged that nutrition education is very limited in the traditional medical school curriculum. This is a glaring deficiency since nutrition is critical to the wellness of every patient at every stage of life. To address this deficiency, MedCHEFS (Medical Student Curriculum in Healthy Eating, Exercise, and Food Science) was developed in 2012 by several faculty of the Eastern Division campus of the West Virginia University (WVU) School of Medicine. Our regional campus seemed the perfect place to implement this innovation because of our small cadre of students (approximately 20 third-year students per year) and the nature of our longitudinal curriculum (our students rotate for six months through Family Medicine/Pediatrics/OB-GYN simultaneously, and then for six months through Surgery/Internal Medicine/Psychiatry/Neurology.)

The first step in developing the new curriculum was for faculty to determine key concepts necessary to lay a foundation for nutrition education. In West Virginia, our biggest burden is related to metabolic disease. Therefore, nutrition and lifestyle interventions for patients with conditions related to insulin resistance (HTN, Obesity, NASH, CAD) continues to be a significant focus in our curriculum. Students were surveyed and wanted practical information to pass on to these patients. The important concept of a "healthy plate" for patients with and without metabolic syndrome was the focus. This included lectures and activities about the nutritional aspects of fruits, vegetables, oils/fats, proteins, spices, and herbs.

Our students needed to learn about nutrition from a broad perspective, as well as specific nutritional concerns related to pediatrics, obstetrics, and geriatrics. We also wanted them to learn the basics of food preparation, and to practice cooking whole, healthy food so they could be informed when sharing nutrition advice with patients in the clinic and the community. We wanted them to learn about public health, food policy, advertising, and mindfulness in eating. Most importantly, we wanted them to practice how to effectively communicate this information to their patients.

MedCHEFS starts with a full day immersion during our third-year orientation week. This includes lectures, video presentations, an assignment for grocery shopping on a budget, case studies, and their first teaching kitchen experience. Our program was initially funded through a dean's grant supporting curricular innovation. With those funds, we partnered with the culinary program at a community college and formed a relationship that allows us to work with their chef and use their teaching kitchen quarterly at a nominal cost per student. There are monthly two-hour MedCHEFS case-based, didactic, and hands-on food prep sessions during their Friday education days, as well as community-based activities like attending lunch with the students at a local public school with discussion afterwards.

The Motivational Interviewing (MI) session involves pre-reading of several articles on the evidence for and technique of MI. A lecture is presented on motivational interviewing techniques, and the students start by practicing on each other. The session ends with a standardized patient encounter engaging a 42-year-old diabetic female who wants to lose 40 lbs to improve her health. The students are asked to use their MI techniques in this patient interaction. Subsequently, they receive feedback from the faculty watching the interview, and also complete a self-evaluation tool when they review their own video after the encounter.

The challenge of implementing curricular change and adding content to the already overwhelming clinical learning in third year is daunting. We made nutrition a priority and used didactic time initially out of the Family Medicine clerkship, and some extracurricular time for the teaching kitchens and community activities. We later recognized that other clerkships needed to get involved as well. As we have started to disseminate the curriculum to WVU's other regional campus and the main campus, we have developed and shared specialty-relevant nutrition cases with each clerkship (i.e. a patient with nutritional deficiencies following gastric bypass in the Surgery clerkship). These cases, and other components from faculty throughout the school, have evolved into a nutritional thread throughout the whole School of Medicine curriculum.

The culmination of the entire MedCHEFS year is a Mini-Med School session in which the students select a healthy recipe, purchase the ingredients, and prepare it as a cooking demo for community members. The students have engaged approximately 100 community members each year with this outreach. Prior to or during their cooking demo, the students speak to their audience about the nutritional benefits of the foods they have chosen to prepare and answer audience questions. They have prepared recipes like hummus, yogurt vegetable dip, kale salad, vegetable smoothies, and one-ingredient banana ice cream. The community response has been overwhelmingly positive, and the experience allows our students to learn while teaching.

A Student Perspective:

As a medical student, I believe that my most important job is learning and increasing my potential as a physician for my future patients. One of my most valuable experiences during clinical years has been the introduction of nutrition and cooking skills. Every month, we are taught a hands-on class by a community chef with the goal of gaining the ability to encourage patients to lead a healthy lifestyle in the kitchen.

Following these classes, we then have the opportunity to practice diet education and motivational interviewing during both Continuity Clinic and community metabolic syndrome support groups (both of which are additional perks of being a student at a regional campus). In both examples, we build relationships with patients from week to week over the course of a year, which provides the perfect opportunity to use our newfound knowledge to help guide patients in making their own healthy decisions. I could feel my confidence growing in educating patients with each MedCHEFS lesson. By the end of the year, I felt comfortable initiating conversations about diet — a sensitive, but necessary topic in today's society.

The MedCHEFS program has provided a unique opportunity for students at WVU's Eastern Division. It has spread to other WVU campuses, and could be implemented at other medical schools, as well. We learn cooking and nutrition from the experts and then immediately apply our knowledge to clinical practice. Because of this program, I believe that we have gained confidence and the necessary skills to educate and encourage patients, especially in making lifestyle changes and healthy nutritional choices.

Summary points:

- It is possible to incorporate nutrition education into the third-year curriculum. We chose to focus primarily on conditions related to insulin resistance because of the prevalence of metabolic diseases in our state.

- Nutrition education should include instruction on motivational interviewing techniques. We accomplished this through lecture and standardized patient encounters.

- Please contact us if you would like to use any portion of our MedCHEFS curriculum materials.

4. Developing a Medical Humanities Course for Students Engaged in Core Clinical Clerkships

Authors:

- Michael P. Flanagan, M.D., FAAFP,
  Assistant Dean for Student Affairs, Professor
  and Vice-Chair of Family and Community Medicine,
  Penn State College of Medicine, University Park Campus

- Sudhanshu Bhatnagar MS IV,
  Penn State College of Medicine, University Park Campus

Questions Addressed:

1. *How might academic medical school faculty design a humanities course for medical students engaged in core clinical clerkships?*

2. *What would medical student's desire most in a humanities course during their clinical clerkships?*

A Faculty Perspective:

Penn State College of Medicine was the first medical school in the U.S. to include a dedicated Department of Humanities. As such, a humanities component is incorporated into the curriculum during each year of training at our institution. Deciding on what aspects of medical humanities should be integrated into the clinical clerkship year of medical school depends, in part, on the design of the overall humanities curriculum. Challenges specific to the initial clinical experiences in medical school can help to inform the content for a humanities course delivered at this time.

At Penn State, the medical humanities thread is longitudinally integrated into the curriculum throughout all phases of the educational program. Instilling a humanistic approach to patient care, promoting collaborative inquiry, and fostering self-reflection are consistent goals of the humanities curriculum. In the preclinical years, humanities instruction takes the form of five specific areas of inquiry. Each area focuses on a specific topic and builds on the content delivered in earlier courses. The areas of humanistic inquiry covered in the first 18 months of study at Penn State College of Medicine include Critical Thinking, Mind-Body Connection, Communication, Professionalism, and Medical Ethics.

Introducing these topics, followed by discussion and reflection promotes an understanding of humanistic concepts that can be applied during clinical encounters. However, the clerkships themselves create the need to process multiple new experiences, such as death and dying, delivering bad news, and interacting with patients and staff in a culture of respect. This transitional time in the student's medical education is, therefore, primed for applying humanistic approaches to direct patient interaction. The third year of medical school in a traditional 2 + 2 program, which is defined by a two-year period of basic science instruction followed by a separate two-year clinical phase, often corresponds to this transitional time. Consequently, in our clinical phase of training, we have offered a humanities small group experience to provide support along with a forum for safe dialogue.

The progression into the core clerkships is a time that many students begin to experience increased stress. Long hours and increasing demands on their time and abilities creates unique pressures that can be both mental and physical. Indeed, studies indicate that future physicians as a whole start medical school with mental health profiles and empathy assessments that are as good, or better than their counterparts in other careers[1]. After starting their training, however, measures of burnout among medical students increase substantially. Burnout includes feelings of depersonalization, in which students become less empathetic and more callous toward patients; feelings of inadequate personal accomplishment; and an overall sense of emotional exhaustion[1]. This has been demonstrated in multiple studies and appears to spike with the onset of patient care responsibilities.

Increased incidence of burnout among medical students is linked to a host of adverse effects for both the students and their patients. Higher rates of medical errors, substandard patient care, and inappropriate prescribing behaviors increase with burnout, as does alcohol and substance abuse[1]. Furthermore, burnout also correlates with elevated rates of depression, anxiety, and suicidal ideation. Indeed, the rate of suicide among medical students, residents, and physicians is significantly higher than that of the general population[2]. Environmental factors for medical students that can contribute to burnout include mistreatment by superiors, constant formal evaluations, and long work hours.

As such, when students begin patient care during medical school, a humanities small group experience can be designed to have a lasting positive effect. Providing a setting where students can discuss their challenges, fears, and frustrations in a non-judgmental and confidential setting with peers and one or two facilitators can have a significant impact, minimizing stress and feelings of burnout. It may also alert faculty members to students who might be struggling with specific issues and provide a barometer of the stress level in the class as a whole. In our experience, two faculty facilitators and one fourth-year medical student matched with a cohort of six to eight students creates an ideal small group humanities cohort. Prompts or triggers, such as asking the students to "discuss a personal stress on a rotation" or "share an occasion in which you observed harsh treatment," can all serve to stimulate an interactive dialogue. The facilitators and fourth-year students may share their own prior experiences and thereby demonstrate empathy. Finally, asking students to briefly and anonymously assess the humanities session immediately after each small group can provide useful ongoing feedback to the facilitators.

Medical schools that are moving away from the traditional 2 + 2 educational program might employ a modified approach to the medical humanities experience. A similar format could be integrated with the onset of clinical rotations in less traditional programs, such as longitudinal clerkships. The benefits of a supportive humanities group could be expected to translate effectively into these innovative programs, as well.

A Student Perspective:

For medical students, a humanities course offered during the clinical clerkship year should focus on three primary goals:

1) Act as a space for students to share their health system and patient experiences.

2) Offer differing and thought-provoking views of clinical interactions.

3) Remind students of the importance of maintaining humanistic behaviors during their clinical clerkships and beyond.

A third-year humanities course should be designed such that students can share their experiences, frustrations, and critiques in confidence and without concern for retribution. When done in a group setting, such communal discussions can provide perspective, demonstrate empathy, and promote individual and group reflection.

In many cases, students at a regional campus will work with the same attendings throughout their clerkship year and consequently many may have similar experiences. The second goal of the humanities course is to validate the individual student's experience, while concurrently encouraging them to appreciate the perspective of their peers during discussions. As such, students can learn that similar clinical experiences may also be interpreted in a variety of ways by different individuals. Conversely, they may also have their own impressions validated and feel supported in the process. This exercise serves to build the student's personal repertoire of humanistic qualities as they expand their capacity for self-reflection and critical thinking.

Medicine is an interactive field and students should be aware that their "work" is derived from the human experience. A humanities course provides a medium through which experiences and opinions can be shared. The ultimate goal is to instill long-lasting humanistic qualities in medical students and the future physicians they will become.

References:

1. Dyrbye, L., & Shanafelt, T. (2016). "A narrative review on burnout experienced by medical students and residents". *MEDICAL EDUCATION*, 50, 132-149.

2. Andrew, L. (October 3, 2016). Physician Suicide. *Medscape.* Retrieved from http://emedicine.medscape.com/article/806779-overview.

Summary points:

- The design of a clerkship-year humanities experience depends on the overall humanities curriculum.

- Instilling a humanistic approach to patient care, promoting collaborative inquiry, and fostering self-reflection are consistent goals of the humanities curriculum.

- A humanities course offered during the clerkship year can promote contemplation, commiseration, and empathy among peers, helping students adapt to the pressures of clinical training.

- Providing a setting for students to discuss their challenges, fears, and frustrations in a non-judgmental and confidential setting can minimize burnout.

- The benefits of a supportive humanities small group can also be translated into innovative programs in a non-traditional medical school curriculum.

5. Simulation Sessions with Sim Man and Standardized Patients to Teach Opioid Dispensing Responsibilities to Medical Students

Authors:

- Aaron McLaughlin M.D.,
  Assistant Professor of Family Medicine,
  West Virginia University School of Medicine,
  Eastern Campus

- Rosemarie Cannarella Lorenzetti, M.D., MPH,
  Professor of Family Medicine,
  West Virginia University School of Medicine,
  Eastern Campus

- Lauren Rover MS IV,
  West Virginia University School of Medicine,
  Eastern Campus

Questions Addressed:

1. *How can we integrate challenges of emergency medical care with education and management of controlled substance abuse in a multidisciplinary simulation?*

2. *How do we give students a practical experience with patient interaction and consequences of prescribing?*

A Faculty Perspective:

Despite growing awareness and education, as well as increased federal, state, and county programs, drug overdose deaths have continued to skyrocket across the United States in recent years. [1,2,3] The word "opioid" is now more commonly associated with words like "crisis" or "epidemic". Third-year medical students from the Eastern Division of West Virginia University (WVU) School of Medicine find themselves at the front lines of this struggle. The majority of third-year clerkship rotations occur in Berkeley County, West Virginia, which, along with four other counties, accounts for 41 percent of opioid-related deaths in a state with one of the highest overdose rates in the country. Our faculty had a goal to provide a comprehensive educational experience for our third-year medical students on responsible controlled substance prescribing and overdose treatment through lecture, a standardized patient encounter, and a simulation case.

The benefits of using medical simulation to fill learning gaps is now well-studied and documented. [4] Lectures alone have never been a complete educational approach and even clinical experiences on rotations often fall short. All too frequently, supervising providers can unintentionally influence the medical students' assessments during clinical rotations. Seeing a patient truly "cold" is almost non-existent especially in the environment of emergency or intensive care. Simulation is the ideal venue for students to be the first responders. In our Patients as Educators Program (PEP) sessions, we combine the useful tool of standardized patients with the controlled environment of high-fidelity simulation. The medical students are first introduced to a standardized patient to practice and cultivate their skills at communication. The patient's primary complaint is pain and they may or may not be looking for controlled substance treatment. This session also includes a module with the pharmacist to go over proper prescription writing for scheduled drugs and how to calculate dose adjustments.

In the Opioid-Overdose simulation encounter, the medical students are joined with pharmacy students and presented with an "unconscious patient". History provided to the learners is limited as is common in the "real world" with only a brief, bystander account along with identification and vitals. The students are accustomed to being able to speak with a patient and take a history to formulate a differential diagnosis, and the inability to converse with the mannequin is often uncomfortable and off-putting for them. Eventually, they come to understand the importance of quickly addressing respiratory distress in a patient with a pulse and adequate perfusion. This reinforces the circulation, airway, and breathing (CABs) of advanced cardiac life support outside of scheduled ACLS programs. Once appropriate respiratory interventions (some means of ventilation) are applied, the students must create an evaluation/work-up, which introduces them to tests such as a finger stick, which is a critical, life-saving test that can be obtained within seconds.

Opioid-related learning objectives include the use and understanding of pharmacokinetics of naloxone, understanding half-life of various opioids (heroin vs. methadone) and how it relates to management, use of naloxone drip and titration to a goal (alertness vs. respiratory rate), co-ingestion evaluation and management, and work-up for sequelae, such as aspiration pneumonia.

While the goal of this module is to equip students with the knowledge and skills to appropriately manage an individual with opioid overdose, many of the learning points have naturally diverted to other topics of medicine and emergency care. One of the great aspects of medical simulation is that the learners drive the educational experience. Even after doing this for several years, students will frequently request a study or exam finding or add something to the differential diagnosis that is unexpected and leads to post-scenario debriefing of an unlimited number of "learning topics". Teaching them to deliver oxygen in emergency situations leads to the discovery that they have not learned the practical knowledge about types of oxygen delivery (i.e. Ventimask vs. non-rebreather). Knowing when and how to administer naloxone results in learning how to address a belligerent or combative patient, which can be particularly difficult in this case.

Learning objectives not directly related to opioid-specific management include differential diagnosis of an "unconscious patient", interpretation of arterial blood gas, treatment of Tylenol toxicity (in the setting of co-ingestion), and the importance and use of vitals to help narrow the focus of differential diagnoses in the critically ill.

This has been well-received by our students throughout the years because of the ideal blend of practical medical management approaches and communication skills development.

A Student Perspective:

Like many rural communities, the Eastern Panhandle of West Virginia has been heavily affected by the opioid epidemic. Unfortunately, prescription opioid and heroin abuse are very common in our patient population. As such, during their clerkship training, most medical students in our program will participate in the care of at least one patient who has overdosed on narcotics. Unfortunately, such emergency scenarios do not lend themselves well to practicing independent clinical judgment and decision-making skills. The serious and time-sensitive nature of these situations necessarily precludes students from taking the lead. Rather than thinking through things on our own, we are often playing catch up, trying to follow the thought process of our attending physician in order to understand why each test or intervention was done. The experience becomes more about passively *understanding* existing facts rather than actively *applying* our knowledge to produce an assessment and plan.

This is why simulated clinical scenarios add tremendous value to the medical education process. They provide an opportunity for students to practice independently generating a diagnosis and plan, even for emergency situations, in a safe and controlled environment, with immediately-available feedback from the observing clinician. In the case of our opioid overdose scenario, the initial information provided could be consistent with a wide variety of diagnoses. In order to narrow it down, students must be able to quickly produce a comprehensive list of possible diagnoses while also determining what history, physical exam, and diagnostic studies should be performed to narrow down the differential. Once the diagnosis is determined (and sometimes even before) students must come up with a plan to stabilize and treat the patient. Being able to practice these basic skills in real-time fosters a deeper understanding of the clinical process and solidifies important concepts in a way that retrospective case analysis or passive study could not.

Confidence with these skills in the setting of narcotic overdose is particularly important for the future rural physician, who may ultimately work in a community with a high incidence of opioid abuse and consequently see such cases on a regular basis. Participation in opioid-related simulations during medical school can help students to become familiar with the management of these cases while also developing their ability to accurately and quickly apply their clinical knowledge. Therefore, simulation sessions focused on opioid-related complications would undoubtedly be a valuable addition to any rural health curriculum.

References:

1. HHS.gov/opioids

2. CDC.gov/overdose/epidemic

3. National Center for Health Statistics.

4. Okuda Y, Bryson E, DeMaria S, et al. The utility of simulation in medical education. What is the evidence? Mt Sinai J Med 2009; 76:330-343

Summary points:

- It is imperative that we adequately educate medical students early in their clinical years on the importance of being good stewards of controlled substance prescribing.

- Mixing learning modalities to include standardized patients, high-fidelity mannequin simulation and didactic pharmaceutical presentations allows for comprehensive education in all aspects of opioid management.

- Simulation can provide multiple learning objectives limited only by the students' curiosity and knowledge base.

6. Restructuring Education using SCORE© in Early Training (RESET): Implications for Developing a Standardized Surgical Curriculum in Undergraduate Medical Education in Rural West Texas

Authors:

- C. Neal Ellis, M.D.,
  Professor and Regional Chairman of Surgery,
  Program Director, Surgical Residency Program, Permian Basin,
  Texas Tech University Health Sciences Center (TTUHSC)
  School of Medicine, Permian Basin

- Valerie Bauer, M.D.,
  Associate Professor and Chief of Division
  of Colorectal Surgery, Clerkship Director,
  Third and Fourth Year Medical Students,
  Texas Tech University Health Sciences Center (TTUHSC),
  Permian Basin

- Caroline Campbell MS IV,
  Medical College of Georgia at Augusta University

Questions Addressed:

1. *How do students feel about the use of the SCORE© curriculum for the third and fourth year surgical clerkships?*

2. *Can the use of the SCORE© curriculum for the third year clerkship standardize curricular content and predict performance on the NBME shelf exam?*

A Faculty Perspective:

The Surgical Council on Resident Education (SCORE©) is a consortium founded by the primary organizations involved in surgical education in the United States. The seven member organizations are the American Board of Surgery (ABS), the American Council on Graduate Medical Education (ACGME), the Association of Program Directors in Surgery (APDS), the Association of Surgical Education (ASE), American Surgical Association (ASA), the American College of Surgeons (ACS), and the Society for American Gastrointestinal and Endoscopic Surgeons (SAGES). To strengthen surgical graduate education, SCORE© developed a standardized curriculum that has been adopted by most surgical program directors. The SCORE© curriculum was intended to be used from medical school graduation to completion of a residency in General Surgery. With graded curricular levels, however, we are interested in determining whether or not SCORE© can be used to satisfy educational needs of medical students during their surgery clerkship.

Variations in educational didactics and direct patient care of "common surgical conditions" creates many challenges towards developing a standardized medical student curriculum for the surgical clerkship. One of the early "Milestones©" for a surgery resident to achieve is basic understanding of "the symptoms, signs, and treatments of core diseases". The SCORE© curriculum describes these conditions as "coinciding with common surgical conditions a medical student may encounter in clerkship."[1] The differences found in unique medical educational settings, such as in rural West Texas, where faculty recruitment and access to medical care is limited, can affect student learning during the surgical clerkship. With this in mind, we wondered if the SCORE© curriculum could be used to standardize the clerkship experience for medical students?

Preliminary studies on the impact value of the SCORE curriculum show that residents in programs subscribing to SCORE© perform better on the ABS Surgery Qualifying Examination (QE) than those that do not. (2) This begs the question as to whether the SCORE© curriculum can promote acquisition of surgical knowledge and improve results on the National Board of Medical Examiner Shelf Examinations (NBME) and United States Medical Licensing Examination (USMLE) Step 2 examination if used in medical school? Furthermore, for our local needs, can performance on these exams be used to validate integration of the SCORE© curriculum in the rural setting of a West Texas surgical clerkship to account for unique differences in educational experience based on our setting?

The challenges to implementing a SCORE© curriculum for medical students were as follows:

1. The extensive volume of information in SCORE© was intended to take two years for a surgical resident to complete. Modules divided into junior or senior levels, and core or advanced topics were felt to be overwhelming for the medical students, even when limited to "junior core" topics. Content was, therefore, focused into 21 "basic topics" and assigned in three topic groups per week, with the last week dedicated to testing.

2. The high cost of SCORE© was prohibitive for the limited requirements of our clerkship program. An affordable trial

subscription was approved by SCORE©, allowing rotating medical students access during their scheduled clerkship, while maintaining all functionalities for the Clerkship Director, including creating quizzes and generating reports of student utilization.

The benefits to implementing SCORE© were:

1. Implementation of the SCORE© curriculum did provide standardization of surgical education for all of medical students. This facilitated the learning of core surgical concepts regardless of the individual student's chosen career path.

2. Learning objectives outlined in core SCORE© modules improved faculty confidence in preparing educational didactics for topics they were less familiar with. These learning objectives also facilitated resident-driven student education through the Teaching Residents to be Teachers (TRTT) program.

3. NBME performance of students completing their surgical clerkship rotation at a regional campus in rural West Texas were comparable to students at the main campus (an urban tertiary care setting). This suggests that the SCORE© curriculum is a good adjunct to supplement surgical education in areas with limited resources when accounting for variability in surgical clerkship experience.

A Student Perspective:

As a visiting fourth year student doing an Acting Internship in West Texas, I found SCORE© to be a unique and interesting curriculum when compared to that of my own medical school and the other medical schools I had visited. The first time I logged onto SCORE©, I was impressed there were so many learning opportunities: imbedded videos and textbooks, question banks, etc. The site was intuitive, user friendly, and contained all the information I could possibly need to be successful in the clerkship. I could access SCORE© from all of my portable devices with quick access to reliable information, which was an improvement over using Google and Wikipedia.

My enthusiasm quickly changed to consternation when I started the rotation. The goals and objectives I was given were reasonable. The number of "core topics" to be covered did not seem excessive. However, when I logged onto SCORE© after starting on the rotation, the total number of assigned modules was overwhelming! Each of the "core topics" had multiple assigned modules. I had visions of the basic sciences during medical school where each of the assigned chapters took an hour or more to read and study. My consternation and dismay was shared by the other medical students on the service who were all very daunted by the overwhelming number of assigned modules.

As the rotation progressed, I came to realize that my concerns were unfounded. The assigned modules were clear and concise. Most of them took less than 30 minutes to complete. Additionally, the more I used SCORE©, the more comfortable and facile I became with the website. While initially, I was daunted by the number of modules for each "core topic", I came to realize that each module was quite focused. Instead of having to search through an entire "core topic" when I needed to answer a question, I could go to the appropriate module and quickly access the relevant information. I also came to greatly appreciate that all of the medical students and residents on the service were using the same information source. I also found the question banks to be extremely useful.

In summary, I am fully supportive of using SCORE© in the third- and fourth-year surgery clerkship curriculum as an innovative strategy to approach goal-directed learning in surgery. However, there is a significant "initial shock" when presented with the assignments. Some of the medical students on my rotation did not ever seem to overcome this "initial shock" and failed to appreciate the benefits that SCORE© had to offer at this level. My only recommendation would be to develop a means of preventing or lessening the initial shock for medical students when starting SCORE© for the medical school clerkship in surgery.

References:

1. The General Surgery Milestone Project: A Joint Initiative of The Accreditation Council for Graduate Medical Education and The American Board of Surgery. Copyright © 2013 The Accreditation Council for Graduate Medical Education and The American Board of Surgery.

2. Klingensmith ME, Jones AT, Smiley W, Biester TW, Malangoni MA. Subscription to the Surgical Council on Resident Education web portal and qualifying examination performance. J Am Coll Surg 2014 Apr; 218(4): 566-70.

Summary points:

- The Surgical Council on Resident Education (SCORE©) curriculum, although designed for General Surgery residents, can be effectively used for medical students completing their Surgery Clerkship.

- SCORE© consists of multiple topical modules that allow students to pursue comprehensive self-directed surgical learning that is in sync with other learners using the same source during the rotation.

- The comprehensive nature of SCORE© can be overwhelming to medical students, so efforts to prepare them for the self-directed curriculum should be included with its use.

7. Developing Electives at a Regional Medical Campus

Authors:

- Stephen Donelan, M.D.,
  Clinical Assistant Professor of Medicine,
  Penn State College of Medicine, University Park Campus

- Kelsie Herring MS IV,
  Penn State College of Medicine, University Park Campus

Questions Addressed:

1. *What points should be considered when establishing a new clinical elective at a Regional Medical Campus?*

A Faculty Perspective:

Establishing a new clinical elective at a Regional Medical Campus can be a fulfilling experience. An organized approach is essential to ensure the success of the new elective. Key steps include the following:

(1) Identifying a faculty member at an accredited medical school to sponsor the elective.

(2) Defining educational objectives for the elective.

(3) Establishing the elective's timeline.

(4) Obtaining host institution approval.

(5) Designating a time for review and evaluation.

Ideally, students should participate in the elective's development. This will ensure they have a committed interest in the rotation. Electives may help students to reinforce an area of medicine where they have had limited exposure or facilitate the development of new skills. It may also assist in determining if the local community is a place in which they would someday like to practice. In addition, with the current shortage of primary care physicians, exposing medical students to outpatient medicine through electives at Regional Medical Campuses may help to address this problem.

Elective rotations can provide an experience that is distinct from a traditional hospital-based clerkship. Hospital rotations often consist of brief patient interactions in which students may only address a single concern. In contrast, medical school electives can be designed to provide the student with continuity of patient care. Our Department of Nephrology developed a medical student elective so students could learn more about managing chronic kidney disease. We promoted continuity through a longitudinal experience, asking students to care for patients in the office, hospital, and local community dialysis unit so they could follow the progression of a patient's illness.

An elective rotation can also promote a team approach to healthcare. Our Nephrology Department promoted this by encouraging students to attend monthly CQI (Continuous Quality Improvement) meetings at a local dialysis unit, where they identified evidence-based treatment goals with the healthcare team. The outpatient elective might also provide flexibility for students to accompany patients on visits to other community providers. In this way, they can learn about their core elective in the context of how it integrates with other medical disciplines.

The practice of medicine in the United States is transitioning to the outpatient setting, where most care is being provided in community offices or even at home. We have a significant need for more students to consider primary care opportunities. Introducing medical students to community-based clinical electives at Regional Medical Campuses is an effective way to expand their medical education and prepare for anticipated healthcare challenges.

A Student Perspective:

Regional Medical Campuses frequently start out by establishing mandatory core rotations as part of the educational curriculum. After the core curriculum is established, the number of courses can be expanded by offering clinical electives. As students, the ability to help create a new elective becomes appealing when scheduling conflicts occur, when there is no current elective in a subspecialty of interest, or when new clinical educators who could provide a unique clinical experience join the faculty. Scheduling conflicts are often more common during the flexible elective blocks of the third year and during the fourth year of medical school, when there are often limited spots for preferred and competitive electives. Furthermore, some students may even find it necessary to create a new elective in order to maintain a minimum number of required credits.

Requests to add a new clinical educator can occur at any time. These requests may originate from a number of sources, such as physicians, students, or deans. Some students may have a greater investment in establishing a new elective than in completing a required clerkship due to a personal interest in the subject matter or a desire to expand specific knowledge. There may be a culmination of factors that lead to the creation of a new elective. For instance, physician-to-student support for a colleague as a potential teaching physician, student-to-student encouragement to tap a physician with recognized teaching potential, and personal interest in a particular specialty were all components in the creation of a Nephrology elective at the Penn State College of Medicine University Park Campus.

A committee established by the Association of Program Directors in Internal Medicine examined the clinical courses taken during the transitional years prior to internship[1]. The committee concluded that electives can be selected to provide a more focused experience in a particular specialty, to gain expertise in specific skills, or to explore other areas in which students may not get future exposure after they enter a residency program. The Regional Medical Campus can utilize their unique resources which may provide opportunities for electives in advanced basic sciences, evidence-based medicine, health systems, medical law, medicine within correctional or mental health institutions, and global health.

To initiate an elective, a faculty teacher is identified, as well as a preferred approach for contact. At the Penn State College of Medicine there is an option to create a "special topics elective" with a standardized approval process. This requires submitting contact information for the student and the evaluating faculty member, as well as course objectives and expectations. Both the student and teaching physician should agree upon the newly-created course objectives and syllabus before submitting it to the host institution for approval and course credit.

Ideally, planning for a new elective occurs months in advance of the anticipated start date. Moreover, the timeline is important as many institutions have established add/drop dates that occur weeks to months prior to the start of a rotation. Early planning allows for flexibility and modifications while concurrently creating course objectives, obtaining signatures, and planning schedules. A proactive approach to time management is critical. It is important to compile the necessary contact names and numbers; identify the start date, time, and location; and distribute this information to the student, teaching physicians, and department administration. It would also be prudent to inform ancillary providers and staff about the addition of rotating medical students to their team.

Finally, it is important to establish a time to review course feedback with the clerkship evaluator. The latter is necessary so that there is a system of monitoring and reporting for future students, especially if the rotation becomes an established formal elective. The Association of Internal Medicine Program Directors asserts that "all electives should have clearly stated purposes, measurable outcomes, communication between host and home schools, adequate supervision, clear work expectations, and an element of reflective practice" [1].

References:

1. Elnicki, M., Gallagher, S.,Willett, L., Kane, G.,Muntz, M., Henry, D.,Cannarozzi, M., Stewart, E., Harrell, H., Aiyer, M., Salvit, C., Chudgar, S., Vu, R. (October, 2015). "Course Offerings in the Fourth Year of Medical School: How U.S. Medical Schools Are Preparing Students for Internship". ACADEMIC MEDICINE, 90 (10), 1324-1330.

Summary points:

- RMCs often start out with mandatory courses. Opportunities for curriculum growth exist through elective clinical rotations.

- The impetus for a new elective may originate with students, physicians, educators, staff, or community members.

- Critical steps in the creation of a new elective include: identifying a faculty sponsor, defining educational objectives, establishing a timeline, obtaining institutional approval, and arranging for evaluation and review.

- Medical students should be involved in the design and implementation of new clinical electives at Regional Medical Campuses.

Community Engagement and Service

1. Creating Outreach Programs for Underserved Populations at your Regional Campus

Authors:

- Madison Humerick, M.D.,
  Assistant Professor of Family Medicine,
  West Virginia University School of Medicine,
  Eastern Campus, Martinsburg, West Virginia

- Ayita Verna, MS III;
  West Virginia University School of Medicine,
  Eastern Campus, Martinsburg, West Virginia

Questions Addressed:

1. *How do you create outreach programs for underserved populations at your regional campus?*

2. *How can you incorporate service learning as a part of the Outreach Program?*

A Faculty Perspective:

Regional medical school campuses can collaborate with local organizations to create outreach programs offering vital services to the local community and a unique educational experience for students. It is important to engage community partners who are able to address the socioeconomic inequalities and diversity within their local population.[1] Goals of community engagement are to "build trust, enlist new resources and allies, create better communication, and improve overall health outcomes as successful projects evolve into lasting collaborations."[1] There are many possible outreach projects including free clinics, exercise programs, and nutrition initiatives.

Service learning is defined as "a structured learning experience that combines community service with explicit learning objectives, preparation, and reflection."[2] By incorporating service learning, outreach programs become refreshing additions to student education. Key elements of a successful service learning experience include active participation, thoughtfully organized experiences, focus on community needs, a rigorous academic curriculum, structured time for reflection, opportunities for application of skills and knowledge, and developing a sense of caring for others[3]. The outreach program, medical student learning goals and objectives, and community needs should be aligned.[4]

Before Planning an Outreach Program:

Determine a specific need within the local community and become an expert about the individuals within the community. This includes elements of culture, economic conditions, social networks, political affiliations, demographics, and history of previous outreach programs[1]. It is important to explicitly define the goals of the outreach project, determine the population you wish to engage, and find key individuals or organizations in your community to help engage the population in a meaning-ful and lasting way. It is also important to decide how you will engage students and what teaching principles you will incorporate into the out-reach experience. Define needed resources to create and sustain the out-reach program (e.g., funding, materials, marketing methods, and person-nel). Recruiting key community members to participate in your program increases the likelihood of success. If research is a part of your community intervention, think about what research questions you have and be sure to gather the requisite approvals before beginning. Speak with your dean or department chair to garner institutional support for your project.

Planning and Implementing an Outreach Program:

Elect a community service chair from interested students within your regional campus class and enlist medical students to brainstorm early in the process to encourage involvement and excitement in the pro-gram. Appoint a faculty member and student to lead the program. Cre-ate a well-developed plan and timeline for implementation. Involve students and community partners. Apply for necessary funding and collect resources from the community partners. Students can learn the grant writing process and communicate with local partners to gather resources. Work with faculty members to integrate the academic cur-riculum and create a service learning opportunity for students. Decide upon a mechanism for recruiting volunteers for your program. Develop a shared marketing strategy with your community partner to promote participation (e.g., social media, websites, fliers in medical clinics, email, mailers, and newspaper ads).

A Student Perspective:

Student involvement is vital to create successful, sustainable community outreach programs at a regional medical school campus.

Community Engagement through Service Learning Activities:

Student engagement in the community comes with many benefits. Community service brings a sense of purpose and can enhance personal growth while giving a sense of contribution to society overall. At West Virginia University (WVU) School of Medicine, students must have 100 hours of community service during their four years of medical school to satisfy graduation requirements. Community engagement allows them to satisfy the requirement and participate in service learning opportunities integrating medical knowledge with real cases. Students collaborating with faculty members and community leaders can promote the development of sustainable projects while simultaneously learn important networking skills that can be applied during their medical career.

Recruitment:

It is essential to have a student leader in charge of engaging peers to participate in community projects. Recruitment and retention of students is critical to creating a sustainable outreach program. Constant communication between the faculty members, community partners, and student leaders ensures that students are up-to-date and engaged.

As Service Chair at the Eastern Campus of WVU School of Medicine, a key duty is to engage students in service learning activities at this regional campus. At WVU, one of the most effective recruitment strategies has been to discuss the projects at weekly group meetings when all the students get together and share ideas. It is also important to offer the students a range of service learning activities with clear goals and objectives. The Service Chair must be an effective liaison between students and the faculty member in charge of the particular service opportunity. At our regional campus, the service chair is also the link between students and the Associate Dean. In turn, the Associate Dean is responsible for sending the Service Chair a list of ongoing projects for dissemination to the students.

The Service Chair sends monthly emails to students and faculty providing an update on every active service project. The chair markets projects to students using social media and fliers in student areas. They also collate surveys to receive feedback on projects that have been or will be implemented.

Examples of Community Outreach Projects Incorporating Service Learning:

At WVU School of Medicine Eastern Division, students can stay engaged in the community in a variety of ways. Examples of current projects include:

1. **Project Impact:** Medical students attend high school sporting events to assist with concussion management.

2. **Teaching Assistant Opportunities:**
   a) **MedSTEP:** Medical students teach premed students at a local University through case discussions.
   b) **Introduction to Clinical Medicine:** Medical Students help teach undergraduate freshman at a local University who are interested in the medical field.

3. **Metabolic Syndrome Group Visits:** Medical students teach comprehensive nutrition education to patients with metabolic syndrome in a group medical visit setting and assist with research to measure outcomes on the markers of metabolic syndrome.

4. **Shenandoah Clinic:** Medical students assist nurses with a migrant farmer clinic.

5. **Good Samaritan Clinic:** Medical students assist with a free clinic, performing H&Ps and precepting with physicians.

6. **Walk With A Doc:** Medical students walk with local community members at the local Farmers Market.

7. **Food Pantry Project:** Medical students teach monthly cooking lessons and nutrition education at the local food pantry, incorporating principles from their MedCHEFs curriculum.

References:

1. McCloskey DJ, et al. 2011. Community Engagement: Definitions and Organizing Concepts from the Literature. In CTSA Community Engagement Key Function Committee Task Force on the Principles of Community Engagement (Second Edition), *Principles of Community Engagement.* pp.1-42.

2. Sell J, and Kanzleiter L. Underserved Community Engagement Through Medical Student Service Learning Projects. Created 19 January 2016, Microsoft PowerPoint File. FMDRL_ID: 5941

3. Stewart T and Wubbena Z. An overview of infusing service-learning in medical education. *Int J Med Educ.* 2014;5:147-156.

4. Stewart T and Wubbena ZC. A Systematic Review of Service-Learning in Medical Education: 1998–2012. *Teach Learn Med.* 2015;27(2):115-122.

Summary points:

- Regional Medical School Campuses can collaborate with community partners to create outreach programs that improve the health of the community and offer service learning opportunities for students.

- It is important to identify a specific need within the community by speaking with key partners and surveying the needs of local patient populations.

- Including principles taught in the medical student curriculum into the outreach projects creates service opportunities that integrate well with student learning.

- Appoint accountable faculty and student leaders for each project.

- Recruit interested faculty and students to participate in service projects to create sustainability.

- Create effective marketing materials to continue participation in the project.

2. Student Leadership in the Community

Authors:

- Heather Cassidy, M.D., FACP,
  Director for Community Engagement,
  Clinical Instructor of Medicine,
  University of Colorado School of Medicine
  Colorado Springs Branch

- Benjamin Fitzgerald MS III,
  University of Colorado School of Medicine
  Colorado Springs Branch

- Justin Holmes MS IV,
  University of Colorado School of Medicine
  Colorado Springs Branch

Questions Addressed:

1. *How can your Regional Medical Campus (RMC) curriculum support community-engaged medical education and cultivate student leadership in the community?*

2. *What degree of community impact can students lead, and what benefits do students derive from such community engagement?*

A Faculty Perspective:

Rationale:

Twenty-first century physicians need more than excellent clinical acumen and effective communication skills to improve the health of populations. They must also recognize important health disparities that can adversely impact community health. Undergraduate medical curricula fostering advocacy, leadership, and attention to health disparities can inform students' civic engagement. The intimate nature of most Regional Medical Campuses (RMCs) facilitates community-engaged education.

Curricular Models:

Medical schools have integrated leadership training for medical students in a variety of fashions. At the University of Colorado, Colorado Springs Branch, we elected to incorporate such training into our third-year longitudinal integrated clerkship (LIC). Named the Clinical and Community Leadership Curriculum (CLC), this curriculum was interwoven within the students' clinical experiences on the LIC and included the leadership competencies of Emotional Intelligence, Conflict Management, and Community Engagement.

Within the CLC curriculum, the Partnership Education Action Project ("PEAK") was created as a team-based, service-learning project partnering teams of medical students with community engagement preceptors at local community organizations. PEAK Teams work collaboratively to assess local community needs and, thus informed, design and implement interventions to positively impact local social determinants of community health. These project teams engage over an eight-month timeframe; their work is mentored based on validated paradigms and published best practices from the social work literature. At the conclusion, PEAK Teams present their work to peers and community partners in an interdisciplinary forum exploring the communities' healthcare challenges and opportunities.

In tandem with the community-based PEAK projects, the students engage in a "Plan-Do-Study-Act" (PDSA) cycle quality improvement (QI) project at their Primary Care LIC site. These projects are complementary: QI in the community and QI in the clinic.

Challenges:

Our group experienced some notable challenges in creating this program. We found that linking new leadership and community engagement content to such traditional competencies as communication skills was a successful strategy. We were mindful of the considerable time required to engage and inform the students' community partners, as well as obtaining IRB approval (when required), for the community projects.

Benefits:

Leadership and community engagement curricula predicated on service learning can be a vehicle for fostering social responsibility, exploring social determinants of health, practicing inter-professional collaboration, and honing students' emerging professional identity. Student evaluations show that the curriculum increased students' interest in inter-disciplinary collaborative efforts and expanded their conceptions of "physician leadership".

A Student Perspective:

Why Study Leadership and Community Engagement in Medical School?

Leadership in the community offers unique opportunities for students to build inter-professional relationships, develop communication and advocacy skills, and make a difference in the community. Partnerships with community organizations fosters student encounters with non-medical professionals. These relationships may build into overt mentorships that impact the trajectory of students' careers; more importantly, inter-professional encounters provide students with insight into how others think about and approach serving the needs of the community.

Leadership and community engagement training hones the students' higher-order communication skills. Students are challenged to understand stakeholder recruitment, resource management, messaging, conflict resolution, and presentation delivery. While the community is the "lab" for practicing leadership in our curriculum, the acquired leadership and communication skills are invaluable when applied to clinical roles and responsibilities, such as facilitating a family meeting or running a successful operating room arena.

Finally, medical students often feel as though their clinical and educational responsibilities hinder their abilities to impact their communities, which may contribute to students' documented loss in altruism and empathy across the clinical years. Collaborating with organizations that are already "making a difference" gives students a chance to contribute to community change. Meaningful leadership in the community can impact professional identity formation and be a wellspring for resilience.

Leadership Projects and Community Impact:

Experiential service learning is an important complement to our didactic curriculum. The following examples demonstrate the variety and extent of quantifiable impact that student leadership has had on clinical care and local community health:

PEAK Projects:

- Designed and implemented a health professions mentorship program for high school students
- Conceptualized community nutrition courses with the local YMCA
- Developed health and wellness workshops for a local youth homeless shelter
- Advocated the development of a medical school curriculum teaching culturally-competent care for adults with intellectual and developmental disabilities
- Assessed local LGBTQI youth's interactions with the health care system

Quality Improvement Projects:

- Designed an intervention to increase naloxone prescriptions for VA patients taking more than 50 morphine equivalents per day
- Increased hepatitis C screening from 48 to 68 percent at a U.S. military hospital
- Decreased faculty "screen-time" by 30 percent via a student-designed EMR optimization
- Assessed the role of health literacy in osteoporosis interventions

Mission Medical Clinic: An Example of Student Leadership in the Community:

A deep dive into one PEAK Project illustrates the potential impact of student leadership in the community. Students championed the development of a local opportunity to volunteer clinical services on behalf of Southern Colorado's most vulnerable patients. A team of medical students collaborated with Mission Medical Clinic, a respected veteran of Colorado Springs' "safety net", to develop a student-led interface within Mission Medical's longstanding operation. Colorado Springs Branch students now provide mentored primary care to adults lacking medical insurance at Mission Medical, and lead quality improvement initiatives on-site. Coordinating volunteers, supervising clinical operations, navigating social services, and finessing the institutional partnership challenged students to grow their leadership armamentarium. Mission Medical has benefited from this partnership through increased clinical capacity, recruitment of additional clinicians, and fresh ideas for systems improvement.

References:

1. Webb A, et al. A First Step Toward Understanding Best Practices in Leadership Training in Undergraduate Medical Education: A Systemic Review. Acad Med. 2014; 89:00-00

2. Blumenthal D, et al. Addressing the Leadership Gap in Medicine: Residents' Need for Systemic Leadership Development Training. Acad Med. 2012; 87: 513-522.

3. Long J, el al. Developing Leadership and Advocacy Skills in Medical Students Through Service Learning. J Public Health Management Practice. 2011; 17(4): 369-372.

4. Sheline B, et al. The Primary Care Leadership Track at the Duke University School of Medicine: Creating Change Agents to Improve Population Health. Acad Med. 2014; 89: 1370-1374.

5. Strasser R, et al. Putting Communities in the Driver's Seat: The Realities of Community-Engaged Medical Education. Acad Med. 2015; 90:1466-1470.

Summary points:

- The intimacy of the RMC offers fertile ground for community-engaged medical education.

- Leadership is a developed, rather than innate, skill, and is critical to the career of contemporary physicians.

- Linking novel content to traditional competencies enables integration of leadership and community engagement training into the core clinical year.

- Community partnerships can complement clinical arenas by serving as the "lab" for training physician leaders.

- Leadership and community engagement curricula predicated on service learning can be a vehicle for fostering social responsibility, exploring social determinants of health, practicing inter-professional collaboration, and honing the students' emerging professional identity.

3. Community Preceptor Engagement and Retention

Authors:

- Vicki Hayes, M.D.,
  Faculty Physician, Medical Education
  and Family Medicine Departments,
  Tufts University School of Medicine,
  Maine Medical Center Campus

- Michael P. H. Stanley MS IV,
  Tufts University School of Medicine,
  Maine Track Program

Questions Addressed:

1. *How might you identify and attract community preceptors at a Regional Medical Campus?*

2. *How do you support and retain these teachers?*

A Faculty Perspective:

Recruiting and retaining community preceptors for involvement in medical student education can be a serious challenge. Several frequently cited barriers include inadequate provision of teaching time[1,2], compensation issues related to productivity pressures[1,2,3], concerns about patient and staff acceptance[1], competing interests among a variety of health professions and institutions for student educators, and reservations about teaching skills[1].

Institutional Engagement and Recruitment:

Valuing and supporting the educational mission begins with the engagement of Regional Medical Campus (RMC) leadership with institutional and clinical leadership at community preceptor sites. Preceptors can be recruited directly, but it is much more effective to engage CEOs, CFOs, and practice managers, in addition to clinical and support staff, in the process wherever possible. A site visit to a hospital or clinic that includes all stakeholders is one consideration. It is important to share your compensation model if applicable. We support primary care preceptors within our system with a small partial full-time equivalent allotment, and time is blocked in their schedules when they have a learner. It is critical that frequent communication is maintained[2], and that all stakeholders are involved in the planning, execution, and support process. During recruitment, it is helpful to emphasize the increased job satisfaction that typically accompanies teaching[1], the esteem in which the community and patients hold educators, and the value of teaching as a recruiting tool. Methods to identify possible teachers include networking and tabling at regional medical society and specialty meetings, recruitment newsletters, recommendations from colleagues and students, and targeting recent residency graduates. Introducing teachers into the process with a smaller teaching commitment (shadowing opportunities, first-year apprenticeship models, brief rural exposures) can prime preceptors to become accepting of a more robust future commitment. Community preceptors can also support an Inter-professional Education (IPE) model that allows the simultaneous inclusion of students from multiple health disciplines who can learn with and about one another.

Productivity and Compensation:

In addition to promoting institutional buy-in for direct compensation and time allotments[4], community preceptors often benefit from faculty development focused on efficient teaching[3]. They can be provided with a series of teaching tips (such as the One-Minute Preceptor) to help incorporate students into busy practices. This can be accomplished through in-person faculty development sessions, webinars, and online modules. Some states (Maryland, Georgia, and Colorado) offer a tax credit to qualifying physicians who serve as preceptors to medical students. CME credits can be awarded under the AMA PRA Category 1 Credit™ for learning associated with teaching. As previously mentioned, some Regional Medical Campuses are able to provide a stipend to their community preceptors or their practice site. Even a small remuneration signals that the teaching support is valued.

Recognition and Faculty Development:

The term "faculty" (instead of "preceptor") is preferred as a way to honor their commitment to education. In addition to bestowing a faculty appointment, engaging community faculty in the promotion process should be considered whenever possible. Access to faculty-related benefits such as library services and faculty development opportunities can be important, as well as including community faculty on committees involved in the planning and execution of regional student education. You can show gratitude with certificates of appreciation and electronic or hand-written thank-you notes. Individuals and practice sites can be recognized for their teaching excellence[2], and this recognition can be featured in local media, newsletters, or emails. A plaque or other certificate that can be prominently displayed in teaching sites demonstrates that community preceptors are a part of your educational community. Faculty development dinners can create important networking opportunities. Finally, it is important to keep these individuals (as well as their communities) updated on the career path of students they have supported.

Other Benefits:

It is always important to emphasize the intrinsic rewards associated with teaching, such as the opportunity to share in the satisfaction of patient care, to be a role model, and to witness student mastery of skills and their successes[3,5]. Medical students tend to be engaging and stimulate teaching, and they inspire educators to stay up-to-date. Finally, from a workforce development standpoint, exposing students to a community practice might prompt them to consider practicing in a similar environment in the future.

A Student Perspective:

Students as a Source of Information:

Students can be a source of new information regarding diseases and treatment, essentially providing continuing medical education for their faculty. This could take the form of a targeted literature review of a patient-specific question, or a more formal presentation such as grand rounds or a morbidity and mortality conference. Students can update faculty on new guidelines or alert them to some of the latest changes in practice. They can assist faculty in their adjustment to new opportunities, such as helping faculty construct tables and templates in a new electronic medical record. Faculty often acknowledge that one reason they continue to teach is the enhancement to their own education that results from working with students.

Students as Contributors to Clinical Practice:

As medical students advance in training, they can alleviate increasingly constrained schedules. For example, a student can begin interviewing one patient while the faculty preceptor works with a more acute or difficult case. The student can subsequently present the patient he/she has been seeing, resulting in a more efficient experience for the provider and the patient. While the student learns from practicing clinical skills, the patient typically feels that they have had a thorough evaluation (as opposed to sitting alone in a consultation room while another patient is being seen). The student can also interact with other healthcare workers in the clinic, and he or she can facilitate workflow by making consultant calls, following up with pharmacies, etc. These learning experiences simultaneously help faculty manage an overloaded work day.

The Student as Shaper of Faculty and Institutional Identity:

Teaching medical students is professionally satisfying at a time when providers face many institutional frustrations. Sharing the intellectual excitement of clinical inquiry with a student and imparting personal wisdom of experience is itself a restorative process. When students follow patients to other non-faculty clinics, they can serve as bridges to these clinicians. During these brief exposures, these healthcare workers become accustomed to and interested in having students of their own, thereby assisting with the process of faculty recruitment. When a facility takes on the identity of being a place of learning, as well as healing, it can help create a more attractive milieu for recruiting physicians to regional medical centers and the communities they serve. Long-term, the relationships formed as a result of this process can be a valuable recruiting tool, increasing the likelihood that the student would return to the practice or the area after his or her training has been completed.

References:

1. Gerrity MS, Pathman DE, Linzer M, Steiner BD, Winterbottom LM, Sharp MC, et al. Career satisfaction and clinician-educators: the rewards and challenges of teaching. JGIM. 1997;12(2):S90-S97.

2. Dallaghan GL, Alerte AM, Ryan MS, Patterson PB, Petershack J, Christy C, et al. Recruiting and retaining community-based preceptors: a multicenter qualitative action study of pediatric preceptors. Acad Med. 2017;92(8):1168-1174

3. Kumar A, Kallen DJ, Mathew T. Volunteer Faculty: what rewards or incentives do they prefer? Teach Learn Med. 2002;14(2):119-124.

4. Denton GD, Griffin R, Cazabon P, Monks SR, Deichmann R. Recruiting primary care physicians to teach medical students in the ambulatory setting: a model of protected time, allocated money, and faculty development. Acad Med. 2015;90(11);1532-1535.

5. Fazio SA, Shobhina C, Hingle S, Lo MC, Meade L, Blanchard M, et al. The challenges of teaching ambulatory internal medicine: faculty recruitment, retention, and development: an AAIM/SGIM position paper. Am J Med. 2017;130(1):105-110.

Summary points:

- Identify the challenges facing community preceptors such as inadequate time and compensation, multiple teaching requests, staff buy-in, and need for improved teaching skills.

- Develop an organized, multi-pronged approach to recruitment.

- Provide institutional-level support through compensation models, faculty development, recognition, and emphasis on the intrinsic and extrinsic benefits of teaching.

- Support student opportunities to practice their skills productively, to share their knowledge insights with faculty, and to invite long-term mentorship with faculty and a sense of an academic home at the Regional Medical Campus.

4. Mutually Beneficial Community-Campus Relationships

Authors:

- Joel C. Rosenfeld, M.D., M.Ed.,
  Chief Academic Officer,
  St. Luke's University Health Network,
  Senior Associate Dean and Professor of Surgery,
  Lewis Katz School of Medicine at Temple University /
  St. Luke's University Health Network

- Kathleen A. Dave Ph.D.,
  Assistant Dean for Student Affairs,
  Clinical Assistant Professor of Neurology,
  Lewis Katz School of Medicine at Temple University /
  St. Luke's University Health Network

- Leah Grandi MS IV,
  Lewis Katz School of Medicine at Temple University /
  St. Luke's University Health Network

Questions Addressed:

1. *How might a Regional Medical Campus benefit the surrounding community?*

2. *How may the community support the regional campus and its medical students?*

A Faculty Perspective:

Lewis Katz School of Medicine at Temple University (LKSOM) and St. Luke's University Health Network (SLUHN) both highly value community engagement and service. These shared values have been an important factor in the success of the Temple/St. Luke's Regional Medical School Campus (Temple/St. Luke's) and the mutually beneficial relationship between the regional campus and the surrounding community. Temple/St. Luke's, its medical students, faculty, and administration have benefited the local community in the Lehigh Valley through volunteerism, educational opportunities, and both direct and indirect economic effects.

The students' and faculty's engagement with the community on the south side of Bethlehem, and with students in the Bethlehem Area School District (BASD), have developed into substantial, long-term partnerships. Health, Education, Advocacy, and Resources Temple/St. Luke's (H.E.A.R.T.S.) is a student-run free clinic, founded by students to increase access to care for uninsured and underinsured Bethlehem residents. Students help their patients manage illness, access preventive screenings, and connect with mental health providers, registered dieticians, and other resources. H.E.A.R.T.S. provides medical students in all four years with another learning environment in which to improve their clinical skills. The clinic, located in the Broughal Middle School's Family Center, is a partnership between SLUHN, LKSOM, Lehigh University, BASD, and Bethlehem Health Bureau. H.E.A.R.T.S. has faculty advisors and physician faculty members who volunteer to precept each clinic.

Medical students have also developed and implemented health education fairs for elementary and high school students. BASD has two high schools — Liberty and Freedom. At Liberty, medical students discuss topics including smoking cessation, alcoholism, drug abuse, eating disorders, sexually transmitted infections and safe sex, bullying, and physical and sexual abuse with high school students. Feedback over the past five years, from teachers and high school students, as well as the medical students, has been consistently positive. Therefore, similar medical student-initiated sessions, initially focused on drug abuse, have started at Freedom High School. Marvine Elementary School serves Marvine Village, a low-income, public housing community. After discussions with the principal, several medical students developed an engaging, activity-based health fair to teach fifth graders about nutrition, good body hygiene, infectious disease and vaccines, feelings and mental health, heart health, and living with diabetes.

The administration and science teachers at Freedom and Liberty High Schools have also implemented an innovative, multi-year, national science course entitled, "Project Lead the Way (PLTW): Biomedical Science." Medical students have been involved in this course since its inception. The student leaders work with high school teachers and medical school faculty advisors to develop activities and clinical vignettes that complement the PLTW curriculum and enhance the clinical, "real world" relevance for the high school students. Other Lehigh Valley community organizations with which medical students have done service projects include: Brain Awareness Week (Lehigh Valley Chapter of the Society for Neuroscience/Dana Foundation), Da Vinci Science Center, DeFranco Elementary School (Bangor Area School District), Historic Bethlehem, Lehigh Valley Zoo, Meals on Wheels, and Sixth Street Shelter. For all health education events, the medical student leaders have a faculty advisor and they typically recruit additional medical student volunteers.

Our regional campus affords community members the opportunity to complete the majority of their medical education, years two, three, and four, in their home region. Prior to the founding of the Temple/St. Luke's program, third and fourth year clinical rotations were the only opportunities for medical student education in the Lehigh Valley. Our Regional Medical Campus also offers early assurance programs (EAP) that allow local undergraduate students from certain colleges to be considered for acceptance in their junior year of college. Applying through the EAP may save college students the time, money, and stress of applying to multiple schools through the regular application cycle.

Medical schools and teaching hospitals have large economic impacts on their surrounding communities.[1] The local community has realized both direct and indirect economic benefits from Temple/St. Luke's, which has both direct and indirect effects on local business volume. This is due to both increased medical student spending (housing, food, clothing, transportation, etc.), and visitor spending. The Regional Campus has also enhanced the community's reputation and contributed to increasing its attractiveness to new businesses. In turn, the community has supported the Regional Campus and its students financially. Individuals and businesses have contributed to an endowed scholarship fund. Thus far, we have provided scholarship assistance to all matriculated students. Businesses also offer discounts to students on expenses, such as rent, food, and clothing. This benefits students' individual budgets and helps them feel welcomed. Based on data from the AAMC[2], we expect 50 percent of our graduates to eventually practice in the Lehigh Valley. Further, we believe that fostering strong relationships between our Regional Medical Campus, its students, and the surrounding communities will encourage and inspire students to practice medicine here.

A Student Perspective:

Our program at St. Luke's offers opportunities for students to get involved both in their education and the surrounding community. The H.E.A.R.T.S. clinic allows medical students to work with students from Lehigh University to offer free medical care to uninsured patients. The clinic is entirely student-run and relies on partnerships with local pharmacies and physician offices to ensure optimal patient care. The H.E.A.R.T.S. clinic benefits everyone involved: undergraduate college students get early exposure to medicine, preclinical medical students refine their patient interview and physical exam skills, clinical medical students develop long-term relationships with patients, and uninsured patients receive the healthcare they need. Additionally, the experience of working with patients and teaching college and pre-clinical students is rewarding for clinical students. The H.E.A.R.T.S. clinic fills a need in the local community and gives students another opportunity for teaching and learning.

Medical students look for every opportunity to give back to the community. Students involve themselves in the education of high school students by presenting information on health topics at Liberty and Freedom High Schools. High school students are more forthcoming with medical students about their concerns and struggles over issues like drug abuse and sexually transmitted infections, than they are with their teachers. This is likely because medical and high school students are closer in age. Medical students also gain experience teaching health topics to non-medical personnel. Other non-medical outreach opportunities include food drives and adopt-a-family gift drives. Participation in these philanthropic drives is high among the student population. Reciprocally, community members are generous toward the medical students. All medical students in the Temple/St. Luke's program receive scholarship assistance through donations by local community members. This eases the financial burden of attending medical school. Some students take initiative to involve themselves in the community by coaching a local high school sports team or through involvement in a local church congregation. Ultimately, these connections formed between students and members of the community increase the likelihood of the student remaining in the region for their residency training or future practice.

References:

1. Association of American Medical Colleges. The economic impact of AAMC-member medical schools and teaching hospitals. Washington, DC: AAMC; 2012.

2. Association of American Medical Colleges. 2015 State Physician Workforce Data Book, Washington, DC: AAMC; 2015.

Summary points:

- Opportunities exist to build mutually beneficial relationships between local communities and Regional Medical Campuses.

- Temple/St. Luke's has benefited its local community through:
  1. Students volunteering their time to promote healthy living and increased access to care.
  2. Opportunity for community members to learn medicine in their community; early acceptance for local undergraduates.
  3. Increasing the community's future physician workforce.
  4. Direct and indirect economic benefits.

- The local community has benefited and supported the regional campus by providing:
  1. A welcoming, inclusive environment.
  2. Multiple learning environments for students to gain clinical, educational, and other interpersonal experiences
  3. Scholarship assistance, student discounts on housing, etc

- Students find that local community engagement enhances their medical education.

5. Developing a Student-Run Clinic at a Regional Medical Campus

Authors:

- Michael P. Flanagan, M.D., FAAFP,
  Assistant Dean for Student Affairs, Professor
  and Vice-Chair of Family and Community Medicine,
  Penn State College of Medicine, University Park Campus

- Christine M. Clark MS IV,
  Penn State College of Medicine, University Park Campus

- Clay A. Cooper MS IV, MBA,
  Penn State College of Medicine, University Park Campus

Questions Addressed:

1. *How can academic medical school faculty help to establish and contribute to a student-run free clinic?*

2. *How can medical and other health professional students establish a student-run free clinic?*

A Faculty Perspective:

Student involvement and faculty support to create a student-run clinic can be approached in four distinct phases:

Pre-planning Phase:

Start by identifying a core group of interested students and faculty sponsors, and decide if the project will be interprofessional, which can increase resources, expand institutional support, and produce a richer learning environment. Consulting with other successful student-run clinics prior to launching your own clinic is advisable. The Penn State College of Medicine student-run clinic, LionCare-Tyrone, was launched in the underserved town of Tyrone, Pennsylvania, only after significant preparation. Penn State medical and nurse practitioner students initially traveled to the Cleveland Clinic to meet with students that had successfully established a student-directed clinic there, touring the facility and seeking advice. Faculty with connections to other institutions can help to facilitate this dialogue. Identifying a community with high need is also important, as areas with current free healthcare services may be less receptive to a new underserved clinic. Faculty that have established relationships with community leaders in underserved areas may help to connect students with potential student-run clinic venues.

Planning Phase:

Start the planning phase by defining services to be offered. Keeping it simple early on will facilitate a successful launch. Considering scope of practice helps to ensure all services are deliverable. Define the types of patients and services that will be seen initially, such as general medical, pediatric, gynecologic, or mental health and counseling. Next, identify potential preceptors. A faculty champion can facilitate the recruitment of colleagues. Moreover, an interprofessional approach will open doors to additional preceptors. A faculty sponsor should arrange consultation with institutional Risk Management to ensure malpractice insurance is provided for all volunteer preceptors and students. Review coverage with institutional attorneys and confirm all requirements are addressed before the first patient is seen.

Launch Stage:

Faculty champions should provide support when needed, allowing students to take the lead whenever possible. By the time the clinic is launched, students should be functioning with relative independence. In addition, access to testing and medications should be considered. Faculty can provide information to guide decisions regarding use of sample medications and CLIA-certified testing, pointing out current requirements to track sample use and storage, and maintain CLIA certification. Clearly defined plans for follow-up on test results can be developed by both students and faculty, and will help to avoid fragmented care.

Sustainability and Growth Phase:

Ensuring ongoing financial support will help to achieve long-term sustainability. Faculty and students can collaborate to identify information on potential grant funding, including institutional, community, state, and federal resources. Faculty relationships with local hospitals and businesses can help to facilitate donations or in kind services, as well. Student leadership can be expected to continually transition as they graduate and leave for residency. Faculty are more likely to remain consistent, providing continuity. Eventually, student-run clinics may decide to expand services, preceptors, participants, or hours of operation, depending on demand and resources. Ultimately, a student-run clinic is an investment in both the community it serves and the students who develop and sustain it.

A Student Perspective:

The aims of a student-run clinic should be two-fold:

- Provide care to individuals with limited access to healthcare.

- Foster a medical learning environment that differs from traditional models and allows for practical practice management experience through leadership.

Assessing the needs of the community:

When starting a student-run free clinic, it is important to realize that a community's perceived needs may differ from the healthcare priorities of the patients in that community. A grassroots community needs assessment is vital. This can be accomplished through a directed survey completed *in person* where you would expect to encounter potential patients, such as laundromats, grocery/thrift stores, churches, or local emergency departments. Based on the results of our community needs assessment, we established a student-run clinic, LionCare-Tyrone, in Tyrone, Pennsylvania, where a significant need was identified. This was 30 minutes from our RMC, but there was already a free clinic within a few miles of our campus that was well-established and meeting local needs. The location of our student-run clinic was determined, in part, by the support of the local hospital in Tyrone, Pennsylvania where a large population of underinsured patients resided. After choosing a site, we decided to initially hold clinics on the first Saturday of each month and later increase the frequency, as needed.

Interdisciplinary approach and leadership structure:

Student-run free clinics provide a unique opportunity to foster collaboration between health professional students. Our clinic incorporated medical and nurse practitioner students from all training levels. A well-defined student leadership structure and succession plan are critical for continued success. We identified two student Clinic Directors to oversee all other leadership positions and communicate with school administrators and the local health system. A Clinic Coordinator was responsible for managing day-to-day clinic set-up and operations. An Advertising Chair coordinated outreach efforts, and a Fundraising Chair maintained financial records and worked with the Advertising Chair on fundraising events. A Recruitment Chair invited faculty and student volunteers to staff each clinic. Student leadership team meetings occurred regularly.

Scope of practice:

We recommend an initial approach that is geared toward the primary care needs identified in the community needs assessment. Specialty clinics can eventually be implemented once there is demonstrated need. Early on, our clinic directors decided not to provide pediatric care, as children can receive health insurance under the Children's Health Insurance Program (CHIP). We opted not to dispense free medications in order to avoid dependency; however, we collaborated with local pharmacies to match regional chain-pharmacy discounted prescription costs.

Securing clinic space, supplies, funding, and volunteer staff:

Keeping overhead costs low promotes long-term clinic success and stability. In our case, the local medical facility, Tyrone Hospital, generously provided clinic space that was already functional, but unused on weekends. This facilitated shared costs and a shared patient referral base. As a result of this mutually beneficial relationship, we were able to negotiate the use of supplies, equipment, and utilities at no additional cost. A free clinic should not take established patients from other providers, but should supply services to those who would not otherwise have access to healthcare. If you provide services for patients who would receive pro-bono care elsewhere, you are saving these existing clinics money also. Applying for local, state, and institutional grants provides an important funding source. Reaching out to potential volunteer physicians and mid-level providers early on is key, as you will need at least one volunteer staff member on each clinic date for student supervision.

Risk Management concerns:

Medical students must work closely with school administrators and Risk Management to gain their support and ensure that all clinic protocols align with institutional policy. This includes scope of service, malpractice insurance for students and providers, and patient follow-up. Because our clinic dates were relatively infrequent, the follow-up protocol for labs and diagnostic imaging was a concern. We opted to offer limited same-day point-of-care lab testing (e.g., glucometer) at the clinic. An important consideration when offering point-of-care labs is regulatory compliance testing of equipment.

Advertising:

Building a robust patient base is exceptionally important for a student-run clinic's success. Traditional advertising, such as flyers, radio and newspaper ads, and Facebook posts provide steady visibility. However, word-of-mouth advertising may prove to be most effective in getting patients to the clinic and also in generating community-wide support.

Summary points:

- Identify a core group of interested students and faculty advisors, decide if the project will be interprofessional, consult with leaders of other successful student-run clinics, and select a community with high need.

- Define services offered, identify preceptors, and consult with institutional Risk Management.

- Identify faculty support, specify how testing and medications will be accessed and clearly define follow-up protocols.

- Ensure a smooth transfer of student leadership by encouraging students to mentor each other for succession.

- Student-run free clinics facilitate interprofessional education.

- Community health needs assessments help identify desired services.

- Defining scope of practice early is vital to sustainability.

6. Community Engagement in the Northern Medical Program

Authors:

- Sean B. Maurice, Ph.D.,
  Senior Lab Instructor, Healthcare Travelling Roadshow Lead,
  University of Northern British Columbia;
  Foundations of Medical Practice Site Director,
  Northern Medical Program University of British Columbia

- J. Quinn Gentles, M.D.,
  Northern Medical Program 2017, PGY-1 General Surgery,
  University of British Columbia

- Paul J. Winwood, MB, BS, DM, FRCPC,
  Regional Associate Dean, Northern BC,
  University of British Columbia,
  Associate Vice President Northern Medical Program,
  University of Northern British Columbia

Questions Addressed:

1. *How can a community trust support student and community engagement in a rural Regional Medical Campus?*

A Faculty Perspective:

A Response to a Crisis:

The Northern Medical Program (NMP) is a Regional Medical Campus (RMC) of the University of British Columbia (UBC) Faculty of Medicine, delivered in partnership with the University of Northern British Columbia (UNBC). The NMP is situated in the northern resource intensive town of Prince George (pop ~85,000), some 800 km (500 mi.) north of the UBC main campus in Vancouver.

UBC Medicine expanded and distributed its medical program in 2004, largely in response to the demands of the Prince George community, which was facing a physician shortage crisis. As the NMP was being developed, leadership at UNBC recognized a need to keep the communities engaged and provide opportunities for healthcare students to have learning experiences across the vast rural geography of northern British Columbia (BC).

The Northern Medical Programs Trust (NMPT) was founded in 2002 with donations from 29 communities and local governments in Northern BC, as well as numerous corporate and individual donors. The NMPT funds a variety of initiatives to support healthcare students at UNBC, including rural elective experiences in communities across the region, rural shadowing, rural partnerships, awards for rural healthcare students and medical residents, and assistance with expenses associated with relocating for longitudinal integrated community clerkships (ICCs).

The Healthcare Travelling Roadshow:

One major initiative the NMPT supports, the Healthcare Travelling Roadshow (HCTRS), is designed to expose rural high school students to the opportunities of careers in healthcare and healthcare professional students to the opportunities of rural practice[1]. This is achieved by an interprofessional group of healthcare students travelling to several small towns over the course of a week, delivering hands-on presentations with a large variety of models and healthcare training equipment.

The HCTRS has been successful in promoting health careers among local students, putting rural communities in the minds of the healthcare students, and in engaging communities in the challenges and opportunities of healthcare training programs, both in the north and across the province. Additionally, over the years we have learned that the HCTRS is a forum for engaging community members and healthcare students in conversations about the challenges of rural healthcare recruitment and retention. It is a forum for sharing and celebrating academic successes with community members, and discussing academic hurdles about which they may not be aware. It provides an opportunity for communities in our region to showcase themselves to healthcare students, and through the accompanying media, to promote themselves to a broader audience.

Student Perspective:

The Healthcare Travelling Roadshow:

As a student from Northern British Columbia and an alumnus of the NMP, the HCTRS is very close to my heart, and I believe it is an initiative that exemplifies the purpose and promise of our RMC. Growing up in the remote Northern community of Fort St. John, BC, I can say that opportunities to explore my early interest in a medical career were few and far between. Unlike career choices in other industries, gaining exposure to healthcare career options is out of reach for many students in rural and remote areas.

On my first day at the NMP I asked how I could become involved with the HCTRS. I knew this was a chance for me to be part of the change that is so desperately needed, and to connect youth from our region with the opportunities they need to become the next generation of healthcare providers. I soon realized that the HCTRS is so much more than that.

Beyond meeting and inspiring high school students and igniting their excitement in healthcare careers, I learned so much from my peer presenters and the communities we visited. Sharing perspectives with those studying in other professions such as nursing, physiotherapy, medical radiography, and more, helped me to be a better medical student and now a better resident physician. Nowhere else in my training did I enjoy such an opportunity on such a personal level. Similarly, by visiting communities around the province and speaking to the local healthcare providers, I have gained an invaluable education in how our provincial healthcare system works and how patients navigate it. Now that I am training in General Surgery in a tertiary center, I can better understand and coordinate the care of my patients who have been transferred from these communities. My experience is a prominent example of how the NMP is reaching back to those communities to deliver on the promise of training healthcare providers for our region.

Longitudinal Integrated Clerkships:

The UBC Longitudinal Integrated Community Clerkships (ICCs) place third year students into communities where they are paired with a family practice preceptor for their entire year. During this time, they also complete specialty content as a longitudinal integrated experience instead of using block rotations[2]. In my opinion, these experiences represent the ultimate in rural and community medical education and are a demonstration of how the NMP is fulfilling its promise to the communities in the region it serves. The advantages of ICCs are well studied: ICC students take on advanced roles early in their training[3], have enhanced exposure and participation in inter-professional teams[4], and benefit from longitudinal mentorship and assessment[5]. My own decision to take part in an ICC was informed by this research and the chance to receive more operative experience in third year[6].

As a clerk in an ICC, I felt woven into the fabric of the community, both medically and within the community at large. The seamless transition between my family practice clinic and specialty services allowed me to follow and support my patients through the continuum of their care. I think this format and environment facilitates a learner's investment in their education to a deeper level and allows them to feel more a part of the greater whole. The lived experience of training in a community setting makes it that much more possible to appreciate the benefits and challenges of providing care in these settings, a major objective of the NMP.

Establishing connections to your community and its preceptors shapes what you hope to achieve in your own personal and professional life. I cannot imagine a more effective means of supporting students to become healthcare providers in community settings. My own ICC experience was without a doubt the best part of my medical undergraduate education.

References:

1. Maurice, S. (2017). The Healthcare Travelling Roadshow. Retrieved September 26, 2017, from http://www.unbc.ca/northern-medical-program/healthcare-travelling-roadshow

2. Fleming, B., & MacKenzie, M. (2013). Integrated community clerkship: Medical education at UBC and the challenge of underserved communities. *British Columbia Medical Journal*, 55(4), 192–5.

3. Hauer, K.E., Hirsh, D., Ma, I., Hansen, L., Ogur, B., Poncelet, A.N., et al. (2012). The role of role: learning in longitudinal integrated and traditional block clerkships. *Medical Education*, 46(7), 698–710.

4. Myhre, D.L., Woloschuk, W., & Pedersen, J.S. (2014). Exposure and attitudes toward interprofessional teams: a three-year prospective study of longitudinal integrated clerkship versus rotation-based clerkship students. *Journal of Interprofessional Care*, 28(3), 270–2.

5. Bates, J., Konkin, J., Suddards, C., Dobson, S., & Pratt, D. (2013). Student perceptions of assessment and feedback in longitudinal integrated clerkships. *Medical Education*, 47(4), 362–74.

6. Brooks, K.D., Acton, R.D., Hemesath, K., & Schmitz, C.C. (2014). Surgical Skills Acquisition: Performance of Students Trained in a Rural Longitudinal Integrated Clerkship and Those From a Traditional Block Clerkship on a Standardized Examination Using Simulated Patients. *Journal of Surgical Education*, 71(2), 246–53.

Summary Points:

- The Northern Medical Programs Trust has become a vehicle for community engagement, developing collaborations and strong relationships between the NMP, UNBC, students, and community leaders.

- A community trust, which was initially developed to provide financial support for healthcare students in northern BC, has become instrumental in connecting the communities of northern BC with the NMP and other healthcare training programs at UNBC.

- The Trust is a highly successful model of community engagement which is helping to meet the healthcare needs of the region. Beyond providing financial support, the NMPT is a vehicle which facilitates interaction between healthcare students and communities, which in turn, encourages those students to return to practice there.

1. Student Services at a Regional Campus

Authors:

- Callie D. McAdams MS IV,
  West Virginia University School of Medicine, Charleston Campus

- Kathleen P. Bors, M.D.,
  Assistant Dean of Student Services,
  Assistant Professor of Family Medicine,
  West Virginia University School of Medicine, Charleston Campus

- John C. Linton, Ph.D.,
  Dean and Associate Vice President for Health Sciences,
  Professor and Chair, Behavioral Sciences and Psychiatry,
  West Virginia University School of Medicine, Charleston Campus

Questions Addressed:

1. *What are the key functions of Student Services staff relative to medical student satisfaction at a Regional Medical Campus?*

2. *How can Student Services at Regional and Main Campuses cooperate to assure both required commonalities and inevitable uniqueness in the student experience?*

A Faculty Perspective:

Medical students experience considerable distress that potentially challenges behavioral health and wellness. This highlights the importance of Student Services in modern medical education[2]. Student Services have evolved significantly over the past century. In the 19th century, faculty and their families supported all student needs. In the 1930s, informal committees on student relations and peer support systems provided all services[4]. Currently, the LCME requires that comprehensive support services be dedicated to student needs[3].

A key challenge for Regional Medical Campuses (RMCs) is the need to establish relationships with students who may be spending their clinical years at a different geographical location. This requires effective behind-the-scenes relationships among deans and student staff across campuses. West Virginia University (WVU) – Charleston, located in Charleston, West Virginia, is one regional campus in a three-campus medical school design, based in Morgantown, West Virginia. WVU-Charleston is a clinical model campus[1] whereby students complete two basic science years in Morgantown and two clinical years in Charleston. The Student Services staff on the WVU-Charleston campus include an administrator and three full-time employees who work closely with the three regional deans to serve 70 third- and fourth-year medical students. The WVU-Charleston deans and Student Services staff begin to build relationships during a day-long team-building event embedded in orientation week at the Morganton campus. This occurs during the first year of medical school and provides an opportunity for faculty and staff to introduce themselves to students potentially interested in future training at the Charleston RMC. This introduction lays the groundwork for a connection between deans, Student Services staff, and students for the years ahead.

A Student Perspective:

In late fall of the first year, WVU-Charleston Student Services staff bring regional campus students to Morgantown to visit with first- and second-year medical students. This event provides an opportunity for in-depth exploration of expectations for regional campus students. Topics include the regional campus layout, how to apply for housing, and examples of social activities found in Charleston. Including WVU-Charleston students in this conversation provides insight into the structure of clerkships, social activities, local service opportunities, and how to become involved in regional campus research

This meeting helps prepare potential students and decreases anxiety about a move to Charleston. Third-year WVU-Charleston students are able to share their experiences, establish rapport, answer practical questions, and set early expectations for future regional campus students.

A significant difficulty for students joining a regional campus can be the logistics involved with the move to a new location. Most students at WVU-Charleston campus live in hospital-subsidized housing. At WVU, there is also a brief period at the end of the second academic year for students to take the Step 1 national board exam as they prepare to begin their rotations. Due to the differences in resident and medical student schedules, there is the potential for some students to not have housing provided during the orientation week prior to clerkships. This combination of factors can be especially stressful. WVU-Charleston Student Services, therefore, takes particular care to coordinate the provision of room and board for those who might be challenged by this situation.

The WVU-Charleston third-year Student Services Orientation includes an extensive tour of the campus and medical center, and an interactive luncheon with current students and clerkship directors. This allows incoming students to ask relevant questions about how to successfully prepare for their clerkship experience. The staff also organizes a tour of the city, the three teaching hospitals, shopping locales, and other hidden gems of the Charleston area. This orientation provides incoming students with an overview of the area and allows them to explore the city and enter the first day of clerkship with confidence.

Once on campus, the curriculum is comparable. Inter-campus meetings and interim communications allow for sharing of notes and best practices between campuses. The WVU-Charleston Student Services team coordinates and attends monthly inter-campus curriculum committee, clerkship director and quarterly meetings with Student Services staff, the associate dean, and clerkship coordinator. This mitigates curricular drift, addresses potential systems issues and promotes a collegial relationship across the different campuses. These meetings also facilitate effective oversight of a complex clinical curriculum.

Regional campus students are often concerned that their regional status makes them less competitive for residency positions than students on the main campus. The WVU-Charleston Student Services team plays an important role in socializing how board scores, residency applications, and match statistics compare favorably with main campus students. Those wishing to pursue competitive specialties can confidently do so from a regional campus. To help students prepare for residency, a series of 'Getting to Residency' and 'Career Counseling' sessions are conducted throughout the third- and fourth- years.

WVU-Charleston Student Services also coordinates with students and faculty to ensure comparable experiences on the regional campus. If courses, electives, or specialty opportunities are not available on the regional campus, Student Services helps Charleston students find comparable offerings on the main campus or at other institutions to ensure students obtain the necessary experience for a successful residency application.

References:

1. Cheifetz, C.E., McOwen, K.S., Gagne, P., & Wong, J.L. (2014). Regional medical campuses: A new classification system. Academic Medicine, 89; 1140-1143.

2. Dyrbye, L.N., Massie, F.S., Eacker, A., Harper, W., Power, D., Durning, S., Thomas, M.R.... & Shanafelt, T.D. (2014). Relationships between burnout and professional conduct and attitudes among US medical students. *The Journal of the American Medical Association*, 304 (11), 1173-1180.

3. Liaison Committee on Medical Education. (2014). Functions and structure of a medical school: Standards for accreditation of medical education programs leading to the M.D. degree. Retrieved from http://www.lcme.org/publications.htm.

4. Sookdeo, S.S., (2016). The relationship between the utilization of student support services and overall satisfaction in medical school. Graduate Theses and Dissertations. http://scholarcommons.usf.edu/etd/6588.

Summary Points:

- Meeting early and often with the first- and second-year students at the main campus improves relationships between Student Services staff and students, and leads to a better transition into the third year at the regional campus.

- Focused meetings in the fall, prior to the clinical year, to review the logistics of moving to the regional campus helps ensure that all concerns are addressed before the end-of-year SHELF and STEP 1 exams.

- Orientation covers the necessary elements from the main campus, and includes other information tailored to the community surrounding the regional campus.

- Regional campus Student Services should anticipate and address physical and emotional needs associated with transition to a new campus.

- Staff must be familiar with the residency application process to prevent delays and errors in communication.

- Regional Student Services deans and staff should model the same level of competence, knowledge, interpersonal communication skills, and professionalism that is expected of students.

2. Career Counseling and Mentoring at a Regional Medical Campus

Authors:

- Jo Ellen Linder, M.D.,
  Associate Professor of Public and Community Medicine,
  Associate Professor of Emergency Medicine
  and Director of Student Affairs,
  Tufts University School of Medicine,
  Maine Medical Center Program

- Kaylee Underkofler MS IV,
  Tufts University School of Medicine,
  Maine Medical Center Program

Questions Addressed:

1. *What do students value in career counseling?*

2. *How are services different between Regional Medical Campuses (RMCs) and primary campuses?*

A Faculty Perspective:

Most students matriculate with at least a glimmer of a specialty choice, but along the way their perceptions change. It is essential to provide information early that helps students learn about career options with periodic reminders of how and where to make connections regardless of their learning site. All Tufts students are assigned to one of four advising communities that include several faculty members. Each faculty advisor, regardless of specialty, serves as a general advisor to a small group of students in each class. Maine faculty advisors meet with their first-year students over lunch during their orientation in Maine before the students start in Boston. The same faculty advisors correspond with their small group of students while the students are in Boston and periodically meet with the students in Boston or when the students come to Maine, primarily during the first two years. The faculty advisors receive a small stipend and some expenses are reimbursed (e.g., food, parking).

During the pre-clinical years, offering informal "lunch and learns" or "breakfasts with specialists" allows for students to inquire about specific specialties and identify opportunities for further exploration. Tufts' Specialty Advising, Guidance, and Exploration (SAGE) program is designed to expose students to a wide variety of career possibilities. Faculty and residents from other clinical sites, including Maine, are invited to participate in the SAGE events. AAMC Careers in Medicine workshops led by faculty advisors with specific training are well received and help reintroduce students to resources where they can probe deeper on their own.[1] Tufts faculty facilitate the Careers in Medicine workshops and encourage students to visit the website AAMC.org/CIM, take the surveys, and explore the materials and links designed to help them determine their specialty career path. As students transition into their clinical experiences, specialty interest group events with residents and faculty are one place for students to find advisors and develop relationships beyond their formal clerkships. Specialty interest groups host events for students in all four years, often championed by our RMC faculty and residents as part of their recruitment strategy. Several physicians find renewed meaning in their own careers by sharing their stories and mentoring medical students. Faculty and residents are encouraged to participate in career fairs for third-year medical students held annually at the main campus, and a few weeks later at our regional campus.

Faculty advisors and mentors play a significant role in a student's professional identity[1] and career path. Mentorships may develop through research collaboration, working together on challenging clinical cases, or when advocating for policy change. We have been able to pair students with research faculty at Maine Medical Research Center Institute during the summer between first and second year.[4] Communication with faculty mentors on the main campus is facilitated with email and video-conferencing when students are at another campus. Students and faculty connect with each other through several free or low-cost video-conference resources, including Hangout, Skype, Adobe Connect, WebEx, and GoToMeeting. The best mentorship relationships are two-way, in which faculty mentors learn and grow with their students well beyond medical school. Faculty advisors may interact with third- and fourth-year students through the residency Match experience, providing advice as students proceed through the application, interview, and match process. Several of these Match advisors are practicing and teaching at the RMC, however specific specialty experts are only available at the main campus.

A Student Perspective:

Selecting a specialty for their future career is one of the most important decisions a medical student will make during their training. While many students may enter medical school with a good idea of which specialty they will pursue, there are many more who matriculate without knowing where their training will take them. For these students, career advising services can be immensely helpful.

What do students value in career advisement? Perhaps above all, students value mentorship. This does not simply mean being assigned a faculty advisor that a student may never meet. True mentors put in the time to build relationships with their students and have a genuine interest in helping their students set and achieve personal goals.[2] In addition to mentorship, medical students value early exposure to the different specialties, understanding their aptitude for different specialty choices, and support in reaching necessary milestones to achieve their goals. Assisting with CV development and personal statement editing during the residency application process are two tangible mentoring roles that students value.

Most medical schools offer a variety of different resources and services that help to meet the career counseling and mentoring needs of their students. These include individual specialty panel discussions, elective experiences, peer mentor pairings, and use of the AAMC's Careers in Medicine resources. Additionally, assignment of a faculty advisor is fairly standard. While this service has the potential to be the single greatest resource available if it leads to strong mentorship, it can also be difficult to implement successfully, especially when distance becomes a factor for students splitting time between a main campus and RMC.

Distance between students and advisors is one of the key differences in career advising that exists between main and regional medical campuses. When students are assigned a faculty advisor from one campus, where they may only be for a fraction of their medical training, the distance can force students and faculty to rely on electronic communications. This style of exchange may promote superficial interactions over development of true mentoring relationships. On the other hand, students at regional campuses offering longitudinal clinical curricula may develop more meaningful relationships with local faculty, simply due to the amount of time spent together over an extended time period. Another key difference in career counseling between main and regional medical campuses is the availability of established career advising resources and services. For example, main campuses often offer more specialty panel discussions, career fairs, and interest groups than RMCs since the former serve as central training hubs for a larger number of medical students.

While challenges in career advisement exist at both main and regional medical campuses, changes can be made to provide all students, regardless of where they choose to study, a comparable advising experience. RMCs can match services to those provided by main campuses. They can host local career fairs or specialty panel discussions involving faculty and residents at the regional campus, or they can digitally stream or record panel discussions that take place at the main campus to make the information available to off-site students. Main campuses should serve as allies and support their regional campus efforts to provide comparable services.

Another way to offer students at both campuses an equal academic advising experience, is to offer local career counseling by pairing students with a point person at each location where they will study. Campuses should combine this effort with recruitment of local advisors who are excited to be involved in medical education. If an attending physician has no interest in serving as a mentor, they should not be required to advise students, as a meaningful relationship is unlikely to arise in a forced situation. If medical education programs embrace these diverse approaches to providing advising support to all learners, students at both main and regional medical campuses may feel greater and equal preparedness in choosing their career path.

References:

1. http://aamc.org/cim - accessed 2/1/2018

2. Wald HS. Professional Identity (Trans)Formation in Medical Education: Reflection, Relationship, Resilience. *Acad Med.* 2015; 90: 701–706. Mentoring article

3. Lee, A., Dennis, C., & Campbell, P. Nature's guide for mentors. *Nature*, (2007);447: 791-797.

4. Maine Medical Center Research Institute Education &Training: Medical Students, Residents, and Fellows. http://mmcri.org/ns/?page_id=160 - accessed 2/1/2018

3. Developing Critical Health and Academic Support Services

Authors:

- Kenny Banh, M.D.,
  Assistant Dean of Undergraduate Medical Education,
  University of California San Francisco (UCSF) Fresno

- Loren I. Alving, M.D.,
  Curriculum Director,
  University of California San Francisco (UCSF) Fresno

- Stephanie Melchor MS III,
  Joaquin Valley PRIME,
  University of California, Davis School of Medicine

Questions Addressed:

1. *What services do students attending a regional campus miss most?*

2. *How is it possible to creatively replicate these services with limited resources?*

A Faculty Perspective:

Our campus has been hosting core clinical rotations and electives for students for more than 20 years. To complement this, in 2008 we began a six-month Longitudinal Integrated Curriculum (LIC), and in 2013 we welcomed track students for the entirety of core clinical clerkships. With students calling our regional campus home for up to two years, the need for augmented student services increased dramatically. Longitudinal students (and the Liaison Committee on Medical Education [LCME]) expect comparable services between campuses. In order of importance, we identified the biggest needs to be mental health support, academic support, and access to primary care health services.

Mental Health:

Although students have university-provided health insurance, our regional campus, like many others, suffers health-access disparities compared with the main campus. Access to mental health services was the most difficult challenge. While the main campus has two full-time psychologists available to students at the student health center, no comparable services were available at the regional campus. To address this, we hired a full-time psychologist, while offsetting salary with a part-time university clinical practice. Our psychologist also provides mental health support to residents and other allied health professionals. This allows adequate time for work on wellness programs and research, while providing counseling services to our students.

Academic Support:

The second area of need, academic support, required a more creative solution. Three full-time educators with master's degrees provide educational support on the main campus. These individuals are available to help students develop study plans and provide remediation. Students frequently came to our regional campus with pre-identified learning issues and established relationships with main campus student academic support services personnel. Previously, these students were often referred back to main campus due to the lack of resources. This resulted in a loss of connection and identification with our regional campus. To address this issue, we partnered with our local state university to sponsor an academic support intern position. This intern communicates with the main campus to execute individualized learning plans and assists with tutoring and study-skills workshops. Clinical credit hours from this position are applied to the intern's master's degree program. This costs a fraction of a full-time position.

Primary Care Services:

Finally, issues with quality and access in primary care services were identified as problematic. Despite having student health insurance, the carrier did not have a presence in our geographic region and, as a result, students were treated as out-of-network. Lacking a student health center, we negotiated with our university practices to accept the student health insurance as in-network. Only providers who did not teach students were selected, to avoid conflicts in the physician versus preceptor/evaluator role.

These creative solutions have allowed us to address our three most pressing needs in student services with high-quality, low-cost models.

A Student Perspective:

Having academic and mental health support available throughout my education has been a key aspect to maintaining resiliency as a medical student. As the first physician-in-training in my family, I felt unequipped to meet the fast-paced demands of medical school. This is something that I realized was not unique to me. Classmates from various backgrounds have demonstrated similar needs at some point in their medical education. Although I have always had the motivation to learn and work hard, having academic services available locally has provided me with skills to effectively organize the large amount of information and lectures that come with medical school. This has helped me to gain control of my studying and academic achievements.

Despite the academic support I received in school and the emotional support I received from loved ones, the grueling demands of adapting to the rigors of medical school began taking a toll on my mental health. I reached out to psychological services for the first time after only the first few weeks as a medical student. Since establishing that first appointment, I felt the overwhelming relief of having this resource. It is wonderful to have someone with whom I can open up, and who understands the harsh conditions medical students sometimes face. It was initially difficult for me to reach out because I felt like I was the only one suffering. To my surprise, there was a three-week waiting list because of the high number of requests for counseling. Using mental health services has allowed me to develop wellness techniques to take care of myself in a field where physician burnout is a constant reality. It is necessary to not only provide such services to students, but also to ensure that there is enough help to meet the often underestimated academic and psychological needs of students.

Summary points:

- When students are at a regional campus for six months or longer, the need for critical student services increases significantly.

- Prioritized student needs include mental health services, academic support, and access to primary care.

- Agreements with local universities and affiliate medical groups can fill this need at significantly reduced costs.

- When local services are unavailable, some resources like mental health may need to be brought in-house.

4. The Challenges of Providing Equivalent Student Support Services on a Regional Medical Campus

Authors:

- William Cathcart-Rake, M.D., FACP,
  Campus Dean, Clinical Professor of Medicine,
  University of Kansas School of Medicine-Salina

- Emily Lenherr MS II,
  University of Kansas School of Medicine-Salina

Questions Addressed:

1. *How can a small, rural Regional Medical Campus (RMC) provide LCME-mandated student support services?*

2. *How do medical students perceive the delivery of support services on the Salina RMC of Kansas University School of Medicine?*

A Faculty Perspective:

As mandated by the Liaison Committee on Medical Education (LCME), a Regional Medical Campus (RMC) must provide an academic program and support services for its medical students comparable to that provided on the main campus.[1] Kollhoff et al[2] at Kansas University School of Medicine-Salina (Salina RMC) reviewed the LCME document *Functions and Structures of a Medical School* and identified 17 elements dealing with student support services: 1) student research opportunities; 2) student safety; 3) library resources; 4) Information Technology (IT) resources; 5) study, lounge, and storage spaces; 6) service learning; 7) interaction with other health profession students; 8) academic advising; 9) career counseling; 10) provision of Medical Student Performance Evaluation (MSPE); 11) financial aid/debt management counseling; 12) personal counseling; 13) student access to health care; 14) non-involvement of providers of student health care in student assessment; 15) student access to health and disability insurance; 16) immunization guidelines; and 17) student exposure to infectious and environmental hazards. Not surprisingly, a student's academic success may be dependent upon how well the institution delivers these support services.

Delivering an academic program on the RMC equivalent to that delivered on the main campus can be challenging, but not impossible. Working together, the main University of Kansas School of Medicine campus in Kansas City and the Salina RMC have been successful in providing the RMC students with an equivalent four-year academic program. Developing the required student support services for a rural RMC can be just as challenging, as resources at the RMC (trained staff and financial support) may not be as robust as on the main campus. Nevertheless, a plan to provide these services must be developed — a plan requiring extensive discussions and cooperation between the main campus, the RMC, and the health center affiliated with the RMC. Working in concert, the RMC and main campus should determine which services can be easily and professionally provided by RMC faculty/staff and community affiliates, which services are best managed by the main campus, and which services will require a team effort by both RMC and main campus.

In brief, the Salina RMC has been granted approval by the main campus to provide many of the required services using local resources. Specifically, we have been able to provide research experiences; develop a safety plan; provide internet library services; create study, lounge, and fitness areas on campus; introduce students to multiple community service opportunities; work with the local family medicine residency program, nursing, and social work programs to provide inter-professional experiences; arrange for healthcare through local providers not involved in student assessment or promotion; and establish guidelines for immunizations and policies to address infectious and environmental hazard exposures. IT services, academic, career, financial aid/debt management, and personal counseling require a collaborative effort between RMC and main campus personnel. Creating the MSPE and providing health and disability insurance coverage remain the purview of the main campus.

The approach one RMC may take to provide required student support services may differ radically from the approach taken by another RMC. What is important is that the best interests of the students are served.

A Student Perspective:

Supporting students on a small RMC such as Kansas University School of Medicine – Salina (KUSM-Salina) requires services that extend beyond the curriculum. Medical students require access to services that enable overall success in the pursuit of a medical degree; non-academic factors, such as student support services, can influence academic success. For example, it is critical for a student to have access to advisors who can help scholars navigate through the process of financing their medical education and assist with debt management strategies. It is also imperative that students are able to speak with psychological counselors about the stress and/or depression that the rigors of medical school can cause. The availability of these resources, among many others, are essential to the academic success and mental, physical, and financial health of all students. The KUSM-Salina campus collaborates with Salina Regional Health Center (SRHC) in providing needed student support services. This approach conserves financial resources and provides the greatest benefit to students.

Educating students about the support services available at the RMC starts during new student orientation. Before classes start, students are informed about the training and skills of each faculty and staff member and the services provided by SRHC. Whether seeking a trained professional in behavioral counseling or a skilled financial advisor, students know which member of the Salina RMC faculty and staff can be approached when a specific service is required. The family atmosphere of the small Salina campus promotes easy and direct communication between students and educators. The added benefit of only having eight students in each class is that staff is almost always aware of the mental disposition and academic progress of each student.

Although the Salina campus does a tremendous job of providing its students with every opportunity and service at its disposal, there can be challenges to integrating student services available on the main campus in Kansas City with those at the RMC. When a Salina staff member's particular set of skills is not broad enough to address the needs of any student, professionals on the main campus are employed, providing Salina students with the same quality services delivered to their peers in Kansas City. Interactive tele/video-conferencing is often utilized in these cases. This provides the opportunity for direct communication between Kansas City experts and the students in Salina, negating the need for Salina student travel to the main campus 180 miles away.

From a student's perspective, specific student support issues that need to be addressed on the RMC include: 1) research opportunities; 2) safety; 3) access to library materials; 4) access to IT support; 5) adequate study and recreational space on campus; 6) opportunities for community service; 7) financial aid, academic, career, and personal counseling; and 8) access to health care. Although all of the above services are important, accessibility to library materials, study space, and IT support on campus are critical because of the enormous amount of time students must dedicate to studying. The Salina RMC provides these services remarkably well. A welcoming and understanding RMC administrative faculty and staff is essential to answering questions and solving problems regarding research opportunities, community service opportunities, financial aid, career choices, academic and personal issues, and access to health care. As noted above, the Salina RMC personnel are approachable, competent, and able to provide needed guidance or refer students to the appropriate expert.

In summary, the Salina RMC has the unique ability to provide necessary services to students using a personalized approach. Students know they are well cared for and the atmosphere ultimately enhances student success.

References:

1. Liaison Committee on Medical Education. Functions and Structure of a Medical School. Standards for Accreditation of Medical Education Programs Leading to the MD Degree. www.lcme.org/publications/. Accessed 23 Aug 2017.

2. Kollhoff L, Kollhoff M, Cathcart-Rake W. Providing support services for medical students on a rural regional medical campus. Med. Sc. Educ. 2015; 25:157-162.

Summary points:

- The availability of student services for a small RMC must be comparable to those provided to students at the main campus.

- Small RMCs are capable of providing multiple support services using local personnel.

- The Salina RMC provides required support services through trained faculty and staff, direct and frequent communication with the main campus, and personalized one-on-one contact with students.

- The key element to providing student services on any medical campus is an approachable and understanding faculty and staff.

F Faculty Development

1. Faculty Development for Community Clinical Faculty

Authors:

- Chad R. Stickrath, M.D., FACP,
  Assistant Dean for Education,
  Associate Professor of Medicine,
  University of Colorado School of Medicine
  Colorado Springs Branch

- Michael Cookson MS IV,
  University of Colorado School of Medicine
  Colorado Springs Branch

- Erik A. Wallace, M.D., FACP,
  Associate Dean, Associate Professor of Medicine,
  University of Colorado School of Medicine
  Colorado Springs Branch

Questions Addressed:

1. *What skills and behaviors are necessary for community clinical faculty to be effective teachers?*

2. *What methods can be used to teach these skills and behaviors to community clinical faculty?*

A Faculty Perspective:

Several distinct steps are important to effectively design and implement a faculty development program for community-based clinical faculty.

Needs Assessment:

Curriculum design typically starts with a literature review and a local needs assessment[1]. As community-based health professions education has expanded, there has been an increasing awareness of the need for faculty development programs that address needs of community clinical faculty.[2,3] These programs improve faculty teaching effectiveness and help recruit faculty.[2,3,4] Topics most needed by community-based clinical faculty include: orienting students to the practice, teaching in the time-limited setting, bedside teaching, providing effective feedback and assessment, dealing with difficult learners, conflict resolution, and seeking help from educational leadership.[2,3,4]

Better understanding of the specific needs of local community clinical faculty starts with a conversation with others who have worked with community faculty. At our institution, we met with faculty development experts in the local Academy of Medical Educators; the directors of the Family Medicine and Pediatrics clerkships, who have considerable experience utilizing community-based faculty; and the director of the urban Longitudinal Integrated Clerkship (LIC) at the main campus who trained faculty to teach in the LIC model. We then met with leaders of local physician groups to inquire about potential teaching faculty and the challenges and opportunities for each group regarding student education. Finally, networking with educational leaders through professional organizations such as the Group on Regional Medical Campuses (GRMC) provides valuable insight into faculty needs, student feedback, best practices, and lessons learned.

Establishing Goals/Objectives:

After completing a needs assessment, it is important to develop specific goals and objectives for faculty as they start working with students. Our faculty must:

- Describe the overall structure of the curriculum in which they are teaching
- Know the goals, objectives, competencies, and clinical conditions that learners need to achieve
- Utilize strategies (i.e. wave scheduling) and teaching models (e.g. One-Minute Preceptor) to efficiently and effectively integrate teaching and clinical care when working with students
- Complete required formative and summative student assessments in a timely manner
- Identify struggling learners
- Avoid student mistreatment

Program Development and Implementation:

Multiple methodologies can be employed to accomplish goals and meet diverse faculty needs. Efficient and timely in-person meetings can help foster interpersonal relationships, develop camaraderie among community educators, and show both individual and group appreciation.

We developed a three and a half hour "Core Preceptor Training" using active learning techniques including small group discussions, role-play, and interactive questioning to implement our key goals and objectives. This core preceptor training is repeated annually for new faculty and is available online for those who cannot attend.

There are challenges regarding community clinical faculty, particularly if they do not receive financial compensation for teaching. To maximize volunteer participation in our program, we:

1. Provide multiple faculty development sessions at different times, days, and locations throughout the community to accommodate a variety of busy clinical schedules. Thirteen session options were provided in the first year and over 80 percent of our faculty participated.

2. Offer Continuing Medical Education (CME) credits and meals.

3. Tailor session content based on physician specialty. For example, surgery clerkship faculty lead a session specifically for community-based surgeons with surgery-specific content to maximize attendance and participation.

Throughout the year, additional "faculty-pearls" are provided by email or quarterly newsletter on topics such as:

4. Teaching clinical reasoning skills.
5. Providing authentic patient care roles for students.
6. Writing effective letters of recommendation.

Program Evaluation, Lessons Learned, and Next Steps:

Similar to other faculty development initiatives,[5] our program achieved high overall satisfaction. Participants reported positive changes in attitudes toward working with medical students and their ability to provide effective teaching and feedback. Subsequent focus groups have identified the need to repeat content and use other strategies such as email or podcasts for delivery.

A Student Perspective:

Faculty development requires significant leadership time and effort. Feedback from medical students is a powerful tool to help develop community-based clinical faculty. Students interact with clinical faculty every day and their input is invaluable for improving teaching performance. Successful integration of student feedback requires active faculty and student preparation and participation. For example, faculty development regarding efforts to provide and receive feedback requires regular and ongoing dialogue between the faculty and students to improve teaching and learning. To promote this process, prior to beginning clinical duties, students learned how to elicit and provide direct feedback and were encouraged to share feedback tips with each other on a weekly basis.

Direct Feedback to Faculty:

During orientation and throughout the year, significant effort was focused on encouraging students to provide immediate, concise, and directed feedback. When students provide meaningful feedback to their faculty, adjustments to the training environment are more meaningful and occur sooner than if provided only in structured faculty development sessions. Through the process of giving feedback, students are constantly engaged in their education and encouraged to reflect on bidirectional elements of the feedback process. Reflection helps students frame how they seek feedback, improves faculty delivery of feedback, and leads to a more productive and enjoyable clinical environment. In communities where clinical faculty may be new to medical education, creating the bidirectional expectation of feedback minimizes anxiety and improves performance.

Sharing Tips:

For students, the most effective way to improve education in the clinical environment was to share information with each other regarding practice environments. Information shared between students ranged from how to phrase feedback questions to tips for integrating into different patient schedule templates. Students take "pearls" to other settings to discuss what training success "looks like" with faculty members. Interestingly, after a year of sharing, students observed that there was less variability in expectations across different specialty practices. Conversations between students are not formally scheduled or structured. An organized setting and process for students to share feedback with each other could, however, improve the dissemination of information to students and faculty alike. This may further improve performance and satisfaction in the clinical setting.

References:

1. Kern DE, Thomas PA, Hughes MT, *Curriculum Development for Medical Education A Six Step Approach*. Baltimore, Maryland 2009, The Johns Hopkins University Press.

2. Langlois JP, Thach SB, Bringing faculty development to community-based preceptors. *Acad Med.* 2003;78:150-155.

3. Drowos J, Baker S, Harrison SL, Minor S, Chessman AW, Baker D, Faculty development for medical school community-based faculty: a council of academic family medicine educational research alliance study exploring institutional requirements and challenges. *Acad Med.* 2017;92:1175-1180.

4. Christner JG, Dallaghan GB, Briscoe G, Casey P, Fincher RME, Manfred LM, Margo KI, Muscarella P, Richardson JE, Safdieh J, Steiner BD, The community preceptor crisis: recruiting and retaining community-based faculty to teach medical students – a shared perspective from the alliance for clinical education. *Teach Learn Me*d. 2016;28:329-336.

5. Steinert Y, Mann K, Centeno A, Dolmans D, Spencer J, Gelula M, Prideaux D, A systematic review of faculty development initiatives designed to improve teaching effectiveness in medical education: BEME Guide No. 8. *Med Teach.*2006;28:497-526.

Summary points:

- Faculty development programs improve teaching effectiveness and help to recruit additional teaching faculty.

- Topics most needed by community-based clinical faculty include: orienting students to the practice, teaching in the time-limited setting, bedside teaching, providing effective feedback and assessment, dealing with difficult learners, conflict resolution, and seeking help from educational leadership.

- Educating students on how to effectively elicit and provide immediate, concise, and directed feedback to teaching faculty is a significant component of faculty development.

- Creating a bidirectional expectation of feedback for both teaching faculty and students minimizes anxiety and improves performance, especially for faculty that are new to teaching.

2. Faculty Development and Scholarly Work at a Regional Medical Campus

Authors:

- Catherine Clark Feaga, D.O.,
  Assistant Professor (Clinical)
  and Chair of Faculty Development,
  West Virginia University–East Harper's Ferry,
  Rural Family Medicine Residency

- Natalie Moffet, M.D.,
  PGY-1 Resident in Family Medicine at
  West Virginia University–East Harper's Ferry, Rural Family
  Medicine Residency and former *WVU–Eastern Campus student*

Questions Addressed:

1. *How can academic medical school faculty at Regional Medical Campuses help to establish and support each other in educational development and scholarly work?*

2. *How can regional campus faculty facilitate development of scholarly work experiences for medical students?*

A Faculty Perspective:

At a Regional Medical Campus (RMC), learning can be decentralized and occur in clinical settings which have traditionally focused more on direct patient care and less on educating health profession learners. Expanding the focus from operations and direct patient care issues to academic development for learners and faculty can be challenging. Leadership should create an educational framework for learners and clinical faculty which provides motivation for academic enrichment and opportunities for faculty to create and disseminate intellectual endeavors. The establishment of a Faculty Development Committee provides a framework for regular faculty education for entire departments, which can be carried out in clinical offices. Annual or semiannual poster day presentations, faculty education days, and retreats can further supplement the development of academic clinicians and provide a catalyst for interaction between faculty and medical students in research.

Based on our experience addressing these issues at the University of West Virginia-Eastern Campus, we recommend identifying a Chair of Faculty Development. This faculty member may or may not be allotted academic time for this role. They should have an interest in providing high-yield, inclusive education for the majority of faculty clinicians, as well as have the appropriate organizational skills. A variety of prospective topics should be solicited from the faculty body and presenters identified among the faculty members themselves, other community professionals, or regional experts. Often the topics range from medical diagnoses or disease states to concepts in pedagogy appropriate for the development of new academic faculty transitioning from clinician to teaching roles.

A physical location for the presentation should be identified, as well. This may be at an educational building or in the conference room of a clinic, or the location may rotate. All RMC clinician faculty from neighboring sites should be invited or connected via video link. It is recommended that time be allotted away from patient care for the specific purpose of

Faculty Development. A financial commitment from the medical school leadership can be secured by freeing up patient care duties for faculty to attend. We use one hour of patient care time and 30 minutes of personal (lunch) time for each monthly 90-minute session. This sends the message that campus leadership recognizes and values faculty academic development, and is willing to ensure that educational events are offered to facilitate this. Periodically, a half-day retreat for more intensive faculty development off site helps foster team cohesiveness and exploration of more complex topics. Faculty development time should be periodic and regular, which will maximize attendance. Schedules set far enough in advance will ensure that patient appointments will be minimally inconvenienced. Rotating one faculty out of session to cover emergencies can be reassuring for staff and patients. The presenter should provide the Chair with the presentation topic and three objectives at least one month in advance so that CME may be secured for attendees.

Once regular Faculty Development sessions are established, expansion of the program can be considered. This framework can even encompass required certifications such as ACLS/BLS or ultrasound training. Faculty research can be supported and encouraged by the Faculty Development Chair or specific presenters who may involve individuals in larger collaborative research efforts available through the university or through state/regional clinical networks (such as the West-Virginia Practice Based Research Network). Progressing towards publication should be a goal for faculty and for students. Our senior faculty make a special effort to mentor junior faculty towards this end.

The culmination of our yearly Faculty Development efforts is the annual "Poster and Research Day", which includes hands-on skill sessions, expert panels, workshops, and poster presentations by faculty and students. This event serves as a natural apogee to support collaboration between faculty and students. We encourage attendance for our evening and Saturday event by offering dinner and CME for attendees. Topics for posters often stem from student-driven interest in a particular topic, an interesting patient case, or quality improvement projects carried out by faculty or residents. The posters are judged by volunteer faculty, and modest cash prizes are awarded to the student and resident winners. Professional presentations and IRB-directed projects can then proceed from topics and activities displayed at this event.

A Student Perspective:

While not mandatory, participation in the WVU Eastern Campus Poster Session is strongly encouraged and billed as an opportunity to display any and all scholarly work to local colleagues. For many medical students, it is the first-ever opportunity to present original research, and the experience serves to build a foundation of scholarship early in training. The participants are encouraged to seek out faculty advisors at the beginning of the academic year and work closely with them to either develop an original project or to join an existing quality improvement effort or longitudinal study. In addition to placing an emphasis on the expectation of scholarship for the rest of the year, the learner has an opportunity to build a mentoring relationship with a faculty member.

In some instances, armed with feedback and encouragement from the poster session, students and residents will turn what was originally conceived as a research display for a local event into a presentation at a national conference or a published journal article. In one such case, a medical student turned a local case report of parvovirus B19 infection masquerading as Lyme disease into an article published by the Marshall Journal of Medicine. In addition to the sense of accomplishment that comes with any accepted publication, the medical student gained valuable experience with the process involved in coaxing an idea from conception to publication.

Summary Points:

- Create a Faculty Development Committee/Chair.

- Establish regular Faculty Development meetings attended by as many of the regional faculty clinicians as possible. Solicit topical ideas, ranging from medical information and skills development to pedagogy, from the faculty body and identify potential presenters. Provide CME credit.

- Expand Faculty Development to foster research among clinical faculty and encourage them to involve students. This may include regional and university networks as well as data and statistical support.

- Establish a *Poster and Research Day* annually where students and faculty can present posters, attend lectures, and experience hands-on sessions, while concurrently obtaining CME.

3. Faculty Development Built Upon the Pillars of Partnership and Collaboration

Authors:

- Darshana Shah, Ph.D.,
  Associate Dean, Office of Faculty Advancement
  Professor, Department of Pathology,
  Editor-in-Chief, *Marshall Journal of Medicine,*
  Marshall University Joan C. Edwards School of Medicine

- Michael Niemann MS III,
  West Virginia University School of Medicine, Eastern Campus

Questions Addressed:

1. *How can we build collaborative faculty development as a community of practice?*

2. *What are the key elements for successful collaboration?*

A Faculty Perspective:

Faculty in academic medicine need ongoing opportunities for development in an era of rapid and continuous change. However, across the country, faculty development is purely elective, as most academic medical institutions have limited resources to invest in their faculty. Budgets are often tight, and there is a growing need to maximize the use of limited resources while maintaining programs that interface with a diverse student body, technology, and initiatives that compete for limited discretionary funds. In this context, collaboration is a powerful vehicle to promote faculty development and an effective way to enhance the impact of institutional investment in faculty. As such, collaborative activities and programs are important to individual faculty and their institutions.

Collaborative Faculty Development Strategies:

Learning communities/communities of practice:

Funding agencies, such as the Gold Foundation, offer grant opportunities to meet and work with faculty across disciplines and at other campuses or institutions. This helps participants build relationships that often continue beyond the life of the grant received. Colleagues can come together to address the shared goal of building a culture of care through such activities as statewide summits that include panels, posters, and workshop presentations. The participation of health care educators and providers can serve as a model for effective inter-professional education and practice. These faculty development activities create conditions that encourage and celebrate academic collaboration.

Support for collaborative research:

Collaboration is becoming a key method of operation for biomedical scientists and clinicians to work together on fascinating and complex questions involving human health. It is also the underlying current of the National Institutes of Health (NIH) Roadmap effort[1]. External funding agencies, such as NIH, are attempting to break down the walls that impede productive teamwork by offering scientists from different disciplines equal status as funded investigators on joint projects.

Clinical and Translational Science Institute (CTSI) funded institutions can develop strategies to promote faculty research collaboration either within or across institutions. For example, some CTSI programs support the research projects of partners who work at different university campuses, but share common scholarly interests. CTSI programs often intentionally encourage cross-disciplinary collaborative research and mentoring. In these cases, faculty development is planned and implemented jointly to maximize resources.

Faculty need-based conferences and workshops:

Faculty development should be viewed as an ongoing need and approached as a long-term, continuous effort. Building effective research teams is not rocket science, but it does come with unique challenges. Effective team members and team leaders must possess a specific set of skills for the overall functioning and success of the team. Team science is a new approach to research, calling for increased flexibility and innovative modes of scientific collaboration. A statewide needs assessment survey to evaluate team science and faculty development was launched by the West Virginia Clinical Translation Science Institute (WVCTSI) Professional Development core, which included West Virginia University, Marshall University, and the West Virginia School of Osteopathic Medicine. Based on the outcome, several faculty development activities were collaboratively planned by WVCTSI. One example is using zoom technologies to deliver webinars on team science methods and effectiveness across various campuses. These professional development events were collaboratively planned and delivered by WVCTSI partners, bringing together faculty from multiple institutions and their regional campuses to share information and enhance research development skills.

Key Elements for Successful Collaboration:

There are four key elements common to successful collaboration: trust, frequent quality communication, shared interests and goals, and well-defined, clear expectations and roles. Trust is an unspoken, but essential component in building a successful community of collaborators.

The frequency of communication is key to improving and maintaining trust between individuals, as well as institutions. Both traditional and social media methods are used for communication; monthly conference calls, newsletters, and Twitter can be used to communicate with collaborating leaders. The sense of shared or common interests and goals is critical for maintaining collaboration. Effective collaboration can be accomplished through a shared vision, clearly-defined goals, and a mutual strategic mission. Ensuring that all partners engage in the decision-making process while maintaining the ability to compromise also contributes to a high-functioning work group. Clear rules and expectations reduce the chance for conflict and help to move joint projects ahead. Finally, having defined rules, procedures, and expectations of work group members is essential for a successful collaborative relationship. Collaboration can stimulate new initiatives and innovation by enlightening faculty on new perspectives, while introducing them to a new disciplinary or institutional culture. Although partnership requires time and attention, collaboration can help us to achieve goals that one individual or organization may not achieve alone.

A Student Perspective:

The keys to successful collaboration (trust, frequent quality communication, shared interests, and clearly defined expectations and roles) are also fundamental to the faculty-student relationship and are instrumental in successful teaching.

From a student perspective, areas that are important in helping community faculty become more successful teachers are the following:

1) Encouraging faculty to provide frequent, high-quality feedback to students
2) Giving students a degree of responsibility appropriate for their level of training
3) Defining learning objectives
4) Eliciting the student's knowledge in an effective manner
5) Demonstrating an enthusiasm for teaching by faculty, and exhibiting consistent motivation for learning by students

Helping students to define exactly what is expected of them in different clinical situations is imperative for both the students and teachers to be successful. Providing specific, actionable feedback frequently (i.e. at the end of each shift, day, or midpoint), can help the student understand their strengths and weaknesses. It can also help define an objective for the student to address weaknesses and make measurable improvement from that point forward.

A student will be more engaged and learn more when they are given more responsibility (e.g. seeing patients individually and putting in orders, as opposed to shadowing). The appropriate amount of responsibility for a student changes throughout the year and faculty need to adjust accordingly and make their expectations clear to students. In order to identify an appropriate degree of student responsibility, as well as give useful feedback to a student, a teacher must effectively elicit the student's knowledge, which can be done by "pimping", discussing the student's plan for a patient, or observing the student in action. While this can be time consuming, it is fundamental to the faculty-learner relationship, and some preceptors do this more effectively than others. These examples highlight the faculty-learner relationship and could serve as appropriate topics for faculty development at Regional Medical Campuses, where teaching physicians may not have as much experience with pedagogy compared to their peers at academic medical centers.

Reference:

1. Zerhouni E. Medicine. The NIH Roadmap. Science. 2003 Oct 3;302(5642):63-72.

Summary points:

- Collaboration is a powerful vehicle to promote faculty development. Create a healthy learning environment for individual faculty and their institutions via collaborative faculty development.

- There are four key elements common to successful collaboration: trust, frequent quality communication, shared interests and goals, and well-defined, clear expectations and roles.

- Look for inter-professional partnership opportunities; identify and cultivate faculty members who are committed to faculty development.

- Build a culture of learning based on collaboration, teamwork, and shared vision.

- Talk with students to understand what is important to them as learners, identifying ways to enhance their learning environment in the process.

Challenges at Regional Medical Campuses

1. LCME Review and Accreditation

Authors:

- Thomas K. Swoboda, M.D., MS, CPE,
  Associate Dean for Academic Affairs
  SUNY Upstate Medical University,
  Binghamton Clinical Campus

- Adwoa K. Boahene, MPH, MS IV
  SUNY Upstate Medical University,
  Binghamton Clinical Campus

Questions Addressed:

1. *How do LCME accreditation standards apply to regional medical campuses?*

2. *What role does a Regional Medical Campus play in the LCME self-study and survey visit?*

A Faculty Perspective:

Liaison Committee on Medical Education (LCME) Accreditation Standards[1]:

The LCME looks at these essential concepts involving the relationship between a Regional Medical Campus (RMC) and its parent institution.

1. Central Authority of the Parent (Degree Granting) Institution

Courses and clerkships need to follow the goals and objectives of the parent institution. The curriculum committee at the parent institution is the only body that can approve a new and modified curriculum for any campus. The LCME does not want to have any RMC developing unique curricular elements on their own. However, that does not mean that courses and clerkships on RMCs need to be identical to those at the parent institution (see Concept #2).

At the same time, the LCME recognizes that RMCs need to have a voice in the workings of the parent institution. The LCME expects to see RMC involvement in all major committees at the parent institution (such as curriculum, admissions, and academic promotion committees).

2. Comparable Educational Opportunity between the Parent Institution and RMC

The LCME expects that courses and clerkships at the RMC will utilize the same learning goals and objectives, same forms of assessment, and same clinical content as the parent institution. The system by which these are delivered can be unique to the RMC as long as student outcomes are comparable to the parent campus. For example, a primary care clerkship may be longitudinal at a RMC and blocked at the parent institution, as long as both clerkship types produce comparable student outcomes. The LCME recognizes that RMCs often have unique resources and strengths that require creative means to implement the curriculum.

3. Comparable Assessment Methodology

The tools and methods of student assessment at the RMC need to be performed in a manner that is as close to what is done at the parent institution as possible. Any differences in assessment that may be caused by differences between the campuses in the delivery of the educational content, needs to be kept as small as reasonably possible.

4. Equivalent Student Services and Inclusive Admissions Policy

Student services need to be provided at the RMC that are equivalent to the services provided at the parent institution. They do not have to be exactly the same, but they do need to meet LCME standards, particularly Standards 11 and 12. The admissions and assignment process for the RMC should be included with the admissions policy of the parent institution. It must include a process for students to request an alternate assignment due to appropriate rationale and circumstances.

5. LCME White Papers on Parallel Curriculum and Shared Faculty at a Single Site

These two white papers are often germane to RMCs.

A parallel curriculum is an educational experience for a subset of students that adds unique competencies and objectives to the standard core curriculum of the parent institution. It can take place at one campus or all campuses, and it requires approval by the parent institution's curriculum committee based on an institutionally agreed-upon educational rationale[2]. The LCME must be informed about any new parallel curriculum. Faculty at a single instructional site may teach from more than one LCME accredited medical school provided that several principles are followed. They must have a faculty appointment, have appropriate faculty development, have appropriate case load, etc. In addition, the LCME must be notified by the parent institution before students are assigned to that site[3]. This policy does not apply to DO or foreign medical students.

The LCME Self-Study and Survey, and the Role of the Regional Campus:

Students, faculty, and staff from the RMC should be assigned to working groups as the parent institution develops its Data Collection Instrument (DCI) and Independent Student Analysis during the self-study phase prior to the survey visit. The final DCI report for the parent institution should be reviewed by RMC senior leadership (i.e. the regional campus dean) to make certain that its content accurately reflects what is happening at the RMC.

During the LCME survey visit, a full day may be devoted to the regional campus. This day may take place at either the RMC or parent institution, and the exact time and place will be known before the visit. RMC course directors and clerkship site-directors, as well other faculty, students, staff, and leadership will need to be available to the LCME survey team regardless of the location.

A Student Perspective:

For US allopathic medical students, the LCME accreditation process serves as the foundation of medical education and lifelong practice. Participation in an LCME accredited program is often a prerequisite to medical licensing, residency, and loan programs[4]. Given its central importance to our educational trajectory, medical students should appreciate how the LCME accreditation standards apply to Regional Medical Campuses, especially if they will receive any aspect of their training in these centers.

The LCME accreditation standards emphasize central authority of the parent or degree granting institution. Moreover, the standards require comparable educational opportunities between the parent institution and the RMC. Together, these two accreditation standards serve to reassure medical students that the education and training they receive from RMCs is sound and fully complies with the curricular objectives and content of the parent institution.

While the LCME standard emphasizes comparability of parent and RMC, there is no requirement for the delivery to be identical. This provides a wonderful opportunity for RMCs to uniquely enhance medical student education. For example, students interested in primary care or community-based medicine may be better served by longitudinal primary care clerkships at RMCs rather than a blocked clerkship at the parent institution. In this way, the student can fully explore their interests over time and within a setting that more closely approximates their future practice. More importantly, this has implications for specialty selection and workforce participation. A recent study found that graduates of RMCs were nearly twice as likely to match into family medicine residencies as compared to their non-RMC peers[5].

For the above reasons, medical students at RMCs should be intimately involved in the LCME accreditation process at the parent institution. This should include proportional representation on the workgroups for the DCI and Independent Student Analysis, and liberal participation in the LCME survey visit. RMC students can provide an honest assessment and persuasive argument for Regional Medical Campuses because they can speak directly to issues of curriculum delivery, strengths, and opportunities, as well as future career goals and outcomes.

References:

1. Liaison Committee on Medical Education. Function and Structure of a Medical School: Standards for accreditation of medical education programs leading to the M.D. degree. 2017. http://www.lcme.org/publications/2018-19-functions-and-structure.doc Accessed November 14, 2017.

2. Liaison Committee on Medical Education. PRINCIPLES FOR PARALLEL CURRICULA ("TRACKS"). 2014. http://lcme.org/wp-content/uploads/filebase/white_papers/principles-for-parallel-curricula-aug2014.doc Accessed November 14, 2017.

3. Liaison Committee on Medical Education. PRINCIPLES FOR LCME-ACCREDITED MEDICAL SCHOOLS SHARING FACULTY AT AN INSTRUCTIONAL SITE. 2014. http://lcme.org/wp-content/uploads/filebase/white_papers/principles-for-shared-instructional-sites-aug2014.doc Accessed November 14, 2017.

4. Sakai D, Kasuya R, Fong S et al. Medical School Hotline: Liaison Committee on Medical Education Accreditation: Part I: The Accreditation Process. Hawaii J Med Public Health. 2015 Sep; 74(9): 311-314. Accessed December 17, 2017.

5. Liaw W, Cheifetz C, Luangkhot S et al. Match Rates Into Family Medicine among Regional Medical Campus graduates, 2007-2009. J Am Board Fam Med. November-December 2012. 25(6): 894-907. Accessed December 18, 2017.

Summary points:

- Essential LCME concepts governing the relationship between a regional campus and its parent institution are:

  1. Central authority of the parent (degree-granting) institution.
  2. Comparable educational opportunity.
  3. Comparable student assessment methodology.
  4. Equivalent student services and inclusive admissions policy.

- Be aware of LCME white papers on Parallel Curricula and Shared Faculty.

- LCME standards reassure medical students that RMC training is sound.

- RMC training may uniquely enhance medical student education and specialty choice.

- RMC students should be liberal participants in the LCME accreditation process.

2. The Grass is Always Greener: Surviving Mergers and Acquisitions No Matter What Your Side of the Fence

Authors:

- Robert D. Barraco, M.D., MPH, FACS, FCCP,
  Chief Academic Officer,
  Associate Dean of Educational Affairs,
  University of South Florida
  Morsani College of Medicine – Lehigh Valley Campus

- Eugene Kim MS III,
  University of South Florida
  Morsani College of Medicine SELECT program

Questions Addressed:

1. *What are the drivers of mergers and what makes them successful?*

2. *How do these mergers affect students?*

A Faculty Perspective:

PriceWaterhouseCoopers called 2016 "the year of merger mania" in the healthcare industry. Countless health systems and medical schools around the U.S. are currently engaged in some type of merger, acquisition, purchase, consolidation, or other similar institutional change. Regional Medical Campuses (RMCs) are not immune to the merger craze. Driving this change in healthcare are several factors. There is a need to control a larger number of covered lives to absorb risk, resulting in the pursuit of population health management or healthcare company status. Healthcare is becoming more of a retail transaction with changes in the insurance market. Inpatient utilization is declining, resulting in decreasing revenues for hospitals that are volume sensitive. There are many types of mergers and collaborations. For example, a medical school could partner with another medical school, such as Columbia and Cornell. In another model, a health system could acquire a medical school, such as Geisinger did with The Commonwealth Medical College (TCMC). Conversely, a medical school could acquire or designate a health system as a regional or branch campus, such as the University of South Florida did with the Lehigh Valley Health Network (LVHN) or Baylor with Scott and White.

Health systems may merge outside of and despite academic affiliations, such as our own LVHN, affiliated with University of South Florida (USF) and Philadelphia College of Osteopathic Medicine (PCOM), and Pocono campus of LVHN, affiliated with TCMC. Medical schools can have more than one academic partner and, in fact, may have many, such as Philadelphia College of Osteopathic Medicine has with LVHN, University of Pittsburgh Medical Center, Reading Hospital, Mainline Health, and AtlanticCare Health System, to name a few.

What makes for a successful collaboration? We gained significant insight from the University of South Florida Morsani College of Medicine (USF MCOM) and LVHN partnership. A unique curricular program at our regional Lehigh Valley campus called SELECT (Scholarly Excellence. Leadership Experiences. Collaborative Training) was created in conjunction with USF. This program is a parallel curriculum focused on leadership and emotional intelligence, health systems, and values-based, patient-centered care. The goal of SELECT is to provide students with the knowledge, skills, and behaviors to transform the nature of healthcare and thereby be agents of change.

In this era of "merger mania," adaptability is essential. Aligned cultures, especially in the area of education, help with program development. Both sides had a shared clarity of purpose/vision and this led to the goals and curricular domains chosen for the partnership program. Strong leadership with a vision of what the end product will look like is essential for facing challenges to that vision. Transparency and good communication as in any relationship are needed for survival, and being 1,000 miles apart makes those elements even more important. Shared accountability when encountering challenges prevents adversarial postures and a negative culture. Often those within the merger need the assistance of outside "eyes" or consultants, as with the TELEOS Leadership Institute assisting the USF/LVHN partnership with the leadership development components of our program. Engagement of employees, faculty, and students to foster an "all-in" mentality smooths the rough spots. Finally, a well-written, formal, affiliation agreement to serve as a resource and guide helps give order and direction. This document must be revisited at regular intervals to ensure relevance and compliance. As a result of this agreement, the USFMCOM – LVHN partnership has a standing Joint Operating Committee that meets weekly for the day-to-day operations and a Joint Affiliation Committee to address larger, 30,000-foot level issues.

Often, when health systems merge with a medical school or another health system, the effect on students is not often a high priority during the "due diligence" phase. In fact, students originally served by either organization may be displaced with relatively little notice. The health system organization may then ask their hospitals to take only those students from the newly merged school. This can leave schools searching for new clinical sites for the next academic year. However, does this always affect the students in a negative fashion?

A Student Perspective:

The nature of the modern hospital system requires numerous practices with various specialties, both outpatient and inpatient. Outpatient clinics are typically spread throughout the region surrounding the medical center. In these clinics, students learn individually from preceptors and the fast pace of ambulatory medicine provides learning experiences through repeated exposure to common medical problems, as well as less common illnesses.

Often, the more expansive the health network, the more extensive the specialties available for student learning. A broad and well-developed health network that results from health system mergers allows breadth of experience. This contrasts to other programs that may have limited options for clinical rotations.

In contrast to the outpatient setting, the inpatient experience is one of cross-pollination. Each hospital campus is a hub of activity, where learners from a number of different institutions work in teams on teaching services together: third-year SELECT students, third-year PCOM students, and LVHN residents, as well as visiting students and residents from around the country. While there may be differences in our educational focus, we have similar robust clinical knowledge. Students may learn new physical exam skills through a peer from another institution.

They become a better student because they are around other students who have learned in different ways. In this regard, students in such a diverse health network can develop and advance both independently and synchronously.

While student groups may not often be considered during the "due diligence" that precedes mergers, as mentioned in the faculty perspective, collaborative training serves as a foundation for our SELECT program. Such collaborative learning is apparent within our educational experiences throughout the wider hospital network. Merging health systems and sharing student pools has served to significantly enhance clinical learning in both the outpatient and inpatient settings.

References:

1. http://www.pwchk.com/en/publications/top-health-industry-issues-2016issue-3-2016-is-the-year-of-merger-mania.html

2. Greeting, G. Key Drivers of a Successful Academic Healthcare Merger. https://www.aamc.org/download/456002/data/keydriversofasuccessfulacademichealthcaremerger.pdf

3. Kirch, D. 2016. AAMC News. 2016. What Does the Future Hold for Academic Medicine in a World of Health System Mergers and Acquisitions? https://news.aamc.org/patient-care/article/health-system-mergers-acquisitions/

Summary points:

- Mergers are the new norm in healthcare and come in several types.

- Merging institutions do not always give high priority to issues regarding potentially displaced students during "due diligence".

- There are key components to consider for a successful merger including alignment, visionary leadership, communication, and transparency.

- Students can receive benefits from healthcare mergers, such as increased breadth of exposure, and "cross-pollination" of student groups.

SECTION 2

Regional
Medical Campuses
in the U.S. and Canada

1. Campus of the University of Montreal in Mauricie

Authors:

- Pierre Gagné, M.D., FRCP(C), MSc,
  Professor of Nuclear Medicine,
  Senior Advisor for Regional Medical Campus Development,
  Campus de l'UdeM en Mauricie, Faculté de médecine,
  Université de Montréal

- Pierre-Luc Dazé, M.D.,
  Clinical Faculty, Emergency Medicine,
  Campus de l'UdeM en Mauricie, Faculté de médecine,
  Université de Montréal

Regional Campus:

Campus of the University of Montreal in Mauricie
[Campus de l'UdeM en Mauricie, Université de Montréal]
Location: Trois-Rivières, Province de Québec, Canada

Institution (main campus):

University of Montreal
[Faculté de médecine de l'Université de Montréal]
Location: Montréal, Province de Québec, Canada

History and Mission:

In 2003, the Université de Montréal (UdeM) had a significant need for new quality clerkship rotations to support its increasingly large medical school class. The Mauricie region, located 100 miles from Montreal, had the worst physician shortage in the Province of Quebec (PQ), and no significant involvement in medical education. Within the Mauricie area there were three medical facilities: the Centre Hospitalier Régional de Trois-Rivières (CHRTR), a 450-bed specialty oriented facility; the Université du Québec à Trois-Rivières (UQTR), a local university with a variety of healthcare training programs, but without medical student education; and finally the Shawinigan Hospital Center (SHC), a 200-bed community-based hospital.

In June 2003, the UdeM and the CHRTR created the Campus de l' Université de Montréal en Mauricie (Mauricie RMC), to deliver the entire UdeM medical school curriculum locally. The initial plan was to start as soon as possible and eventually associate with the Université du Québec Trois-Rivières and the Shawinigan Hospital Center. At least one family medicine residency training program would be created, and in addition, optional rotations in basic specialties would be highly promoted. Leaders saw medical education as a means to attract and retain physicians in the Mauricie region, and hoped it would permanently solve the shortage of physicians there.

In August 2004, the first medical students started their pre-medical year, provided through the Université du Québec à Trois-Rivières. A medical teaching building was to be built and integrated into the Centre Hospitalier Régional de Trois-Rivières, where small group discussions, clinical skills sessions and a variety of lectures would be provided, making it the heart of the Regional Medical Campus (RMC). Accreditation was granted, allowing first-year medical students to start in August 2005.

Structure, Governance and Funding:

The Université du Québec à Trois-Rivières provides instruction for the pre-medical year in collaboration with the Université de Montréal (UdeM). All other academic activity is under the UdeM authority. Small group sessions, simulation courses, and some of the formal lectures are provided at the Medical Teaching Building (MTB). Clinical small group sessions are taught at the CHRTR and the SHC. All mandatory clinical clerkships are offered at the RMC. Hence, a medical student could go through the whole curriculum without leaving the regional campus, if desired. Optional clerkships are available outside the regional campus. Two Université de Montréal affiliated family medicine residency training programs are also present and provide a continuous supply of family physicians to the Mauricie region. Funding comes from the provincial government through the Healthcare and Education Ministries. Philanthropic donations provided additional financial support at the beginning, including a $1 million grant from the CHRTR foundation to help in building the MTB. Annual tuition is extremely low compared to the United States. A regional dean supervises RMC activities and budget. The Mauricie regional campus is interconnected with various UdeM academic committees. At their graduation, students from the regional medical campus receive the same Université de Montréal diploma as students educated at the main Montreal campus.

Student Body:

Every year, 32 students are admitted at the pre-medical year level. Most of them come directly from community college, with the majority being 19 years old. An additional eight healthcare related graduate students are added annually at the first year of the medical program, for a total of 40 students per year. Hence, a total of 192 undergraduate students attend the Mauricie RMC. The pre-medical year and the four-year medical curriculum are provided in French at this campus. Nearly 100 percent of the Mauricie regional campus medical students come from the Province of Quebec, and about one-third of these students originally come from the Mauricie region. Student admission is managed centrally, and once admitted, these students must choose between the Montreal campus and Mauricie Regional Campus.

Historically, 40 to 70 percent of them continue into a family medicine residency. A distinct regional campus chapter of the central campus medical student association was created in 2004 and its role has been pivotal in regional campus development.

Curriculum:

Academic oversight is managed by the Université de Montréal centrally, with a copy-paste formula: the same program, academic activities, and evaluations are provided simultaneously according to the same guidelines. The process is facilitated by the appointment of local co-directors for each academic activity (clerkship, small group sessions, etc.). Local physicians are trained in how to teach by the UdeM team. To address initial student concerns about the quality and comparability of the medical education delivered at the regional campus, comparative scores between the two campuses were closely monitored and made public at critical points in the early development of the regional campus. No significant differences were observed.

Residency admission comparability was addressed through mandatory appointment of one regional campus clinical faculty member on each speciality's residency admissions committee. Data has shown that many regional campus students were admitted into very competitive training programs. A longitudinal integrated clerkship focused on promoting family medicine, and subsequently continuity of care was started a few years ago. A highly rated optional rotation was created for both the Mauricie and Montreal campuses' for medical students to attend the Université du Québec à Trois-Rivières anatomy plastination program.

Unique Characteristics:

From 2004 to 2009, the Université du Québec à Trois-Rivières (UQTR) hosted curricular activities and provided for student services. Although medical students were Université de Montréal students, they were registered at the UQTR as exchange students, treated as genuine UQTR students and utilized comfortable rented classrooms at the UQTR. Delayed construction of the MTB caused overcrowding in temporary in-hospital teaching spaces for mandatory clinical activities. This caused some anger at times among the first cohort of medical students, as they trained in each academic year and participated in the design of the MTB, but never had the chance to occupy it.

The most challenging situation was the inter-campus transfer policy. To prevent loss of the student population from the Mauricie regional campus to the Montreal main campus, newly admitted medical students were required to sign a contract stating they would not ask for an intercampus transfer. Nevertheless, five students did request a transfer in the very beginning. This led to a challenging visit and report from the accreditation committee. Following this, transfers were granted for the first cohort of students and the tension inside this cohort quickly abated.

Medical students quickly became local media sweethearts as they ultimately represented hope for better healthcare access in the region. They also became part of the political landscape, felt empowered to contribute their creativity to the initiative and expressed strong leadership abilities in problem-solving. Their determination changed the original vision of the Mauricie campus as they contributed to its growth and development.

Accomplishments:

Joining forces from different universities and medical centers paved the way to start the Mauricie RMC within 14 months and minimized political resistance from other competitive stakeholders. The positive publicity associated with this accomplishment increased the Mauricie campus's attractiveness for all physicians across Quebec. These factors led to spectacularly successful recruiting of new physicians in the Mauricie region, such that many from the first medical student cohort were never able to practice at the regional campus, as clinical positions were filled early on.

The Centre Hospitalier Régional de Trois-Rivières (CHRTR) was granted university-teaching hospital status, which brought major benefits for the population, such as a regional coronary angioplasty service. The CHRTR and the Shawinigan Hospital Center, through multiple government driven mergers, became the biggest clinical healthcare network in the Province of Quebec. With this development came other challenges: the new merged institution includes the whole Mauricie region and another region affiliated with a different medical school. The historic coalition has to be updated, governance issues have to be completely re-engineered and the medical teaching building has become too small.

Future Plans:

Research is still in its early stages at the Mauricie RMC, but significant progress has been made. The challenge of keeping the physicians involved in medical education is complicated by new Quebec government regulations about physician's minimal clinical performance objectives, which translates into lesser availability for physicians to teach. Integration of the regional campus into the newly created mammoth healthcare network will demand patience and perseverance.

2. Des Moines Branch Campus, University of Iowa Carver College of Medicine

Author:

* Steven R. Craig, M.D.,
  Assistant Dean for Student Affairs and Curriculum,
  Adjunct Clinical Professor of Medicine,
  Des Moines Branch Campus,
  University of Iowa Carver College of Medicine

Regional Campus:

Des Moines Branch Campus,
University of Iowa Carver College of Medicine
Location: Des Moines, Iowa

Institution (main campus):

University of Iowa Carver College of Medicine
Location: Iowa City, Iowa

History and Mission:

In 1993, five Des Moines teaching hospitals signed an agreement to unilaterally affiliate with the University of Iowa for undergraduate and graduate medical education in Des Moines. These hospitals include Blank Children's Hospital, Iowa Lutheran Hospital, Iowa Methodist Medical Center, Broadlawns Medical Center, and the Veterans Affairs

Central Iowa Healthcare System. The affiliation agreement sought to strengthen and expand the medical education efforts at each of the affiliated Des Moines teaching hospitals. This included combining resources, increasing collaboration, pursuing common faculty development programming, and facilitating resident rotations between residency programs and hospitals. There was also a plan to increase training opportunities for University of Iowa College of Medicine students in Des Moines and to better coordinate training of University of Iowa resident physicians at Des Moines teaching hospitals.

In 2008, the Liaison Committee for Medical Education (LCME) recognized Des Moines as an official branch campus of the Carver College of Medicine. Since then, 24 students from the Carver College of Medicine have been selected each year to complete the entire year of core clinical clerkship training at the Des Moines Branch Campus.

A new long-term agreement to support the Des Moines Branch Campus was completed and signed by all parties in July 2011. Steven Craig, M.D. was then appointed an Assistant Dean for Student Affairs and Curriculum in the University of Iowa Carver College of Medicine, with specific oversight of the Des Moines Branch Campus.

Structure, Governance, and Funding:

The Branch Campus represents a unilateral affiliation between five Des Moines teaching hospitals that are part of the Des Moines Area Medical Education Consortium and the University of Iowa. The Consortium Board of Directors governing the branch campus includes the Chief Executive Officers of the Des Moines teaching hospitals, the Chief Executive Officer of the University of Iowa Hospitals and Clinics, and the Dean of the University of Iowa Carver College of Medicine. Additionally, the Board of Directors includes a physician educational leader from each of the Des Moines member teaching hospitals, the Senior Associate Dean for Medical Education, and the Associate Dean for Graduate Medical Education for the Carver College of Medicine.

Oversight of the branch campus is provided by the Assistant Dean for Student Affairs and Curriculum (Des Moines Branch Campus) in Des Moines who reports to the Senior Associate Dean for Medical Education at the main campus in Iowa City.

Financial support for the branch campus is provided jointly by the participating Des Moines teaching hospitals and the University of Iowa. A yearly budget is set which determines the annual contribution needed from the Des Moines member hospitals and the University of Iowa.

Student Body:

Annually, 24 students from the University of Iowa Carver College of Medicine are recruited to complete the entire core clerkship year at the Des Moines Branch Campus. There is additional capacity beyond this for most of the Des Moines core clerkships. Typically, between 30 to 40 students complete parts of their core clerkship training in Des Moines. Students choose Des Moines for the following reasons: larger community size, increased patient diversity, smaller student numbers that allow for more personal attention and greater opportunities for procedures, and a strong record of academic success.

There are additional opportunities for students to complete much of their advanced pathway training in Des Moines. Emergency medicine, critical care, specialty sub-internships, and advanced electives are available in Des Moines. Up to 40 to 50 students complete large parts of their advanced pathway training at the Des Moines Branch Campus.

Curriculum:

Core clerkship training experiences are organized in 12-week modules. Students complete blocks of Inpatient Internal Medicine/Pediatrics, General Surgery/Obstetrics-Gynecology, Neurology/Psychiatry, and an Ambulatory Practice module that includes Family Medicine and outpatient internal medicine. The curriculum is identical to the main campus.

Unique Characteristics:

There are additional educational experiences available to students at the Des Moines Branch Campus. These include Advanced Cardiac Life Support training at the start of the core clerkship year, and regular use of a state-of-the-art Simulation Center. All students complete moderate sedation training, several procedure labs (suturing, airway management, bedside ultrasound training, etc.), and supplemental evidence-based clinical practice instruction. Each class of students elects a leadership council to work with branch campus leaders for planning of extracurricular social, cultural, recreational, and service activities.

Accomplishments and Challenges:

Academic accomplishments of students at the Des Moines Branch Campus are equal or superior to students at the main campus. Clinical research opportunities available in Des Moines have led to student presentations at regional and national meetings and several publications in peer-reviewed medical literature.

A major challenge for the Des Moines Branch Campus is recruiting students. This is expensive and time consuming. Every student who trains in Des Moines does so voluntarily. The recruiting process has been made easier by enlisting current students to recruit new students for the incoming class.

Future Plans:

Short-term plans include developing a health policy and advocacy track. Long-term plans include developing a free-standing educational facility to provide space for student support services, classrooms, conference rooms, administrative offices, and simulation activities.

3. Indiana University School of Medicine

Author:

- Peter M. Nalin, M.D., FAAFP,
  Associate Professor of Clinical Family Medicine
  Associate Dean and Interim Director,
  Medical Sciences Program,
  Indiana University School of Medicine Bloomington;
  Senior Associate Dean for Education Expansion,
  Indiana University School of Medicine;
  Associate Vice President for University Clinical Affairs,
  Indiana University

Regional Campus:

Indiana University School of Medicine Bloomington
Location: Bloomington, Indiana

Institution (main campus):

Indiana University School of Medicine
Location: Indianapolis, Indiana

History and Mission:

Indiana University (IU) was founded in 1820, four years after Indiana statehood. In 1903, the Indiana University School of Medicine originated at Bloomington, Indiana. By 1908, the Indiana legislature resolved the competition between two universities, IU and Purdue, by granting the charter for a school of medicine to Indiana University. In the early 20th century, the medical curriculum provided clinical experience rooted in the scientific medical sciences, consistent with best practices endorsed by Abraham Flexner in 1910. The Indiana University School of Medicine combined the university educational affiliation at Bloomington with clinical rotations at hospitals in Indianapolis. By the mid-20th century, the IU School of Medicine moved 55 miles (88 km) from Bloomington to Indianapolis, where medicine aligned with population growth, sub-specialization, and biomedical research in Indiana.

In the 1960s, the state of Indiana created an innovative statewide system of distributed medical education, the first of its kind in the United States. This statewide approach settled prior calls for the establishment of a second medical school in that era. The statewide array of regional medical campuses also planned to alleviate the relative lack of physicians in rural and other non-metropolitan areas. In addition to Indianapolis, eight regional medical campuses comprised the statewide system across Indiana, at or near existing collegiate campuses both within and beyond the expansive Indiana University system. This statewide system of medical education enjoys broad public support and consistent legislative support. In response to AAMC projections of a physician shortage, Indiana University received LCME approval to expand its entering class of 280 students by 30 percent, becoming the largest allopathic medical school in the United States with an entering class of 364 medical students per year. Approximately two-thirds of the medical school class begins medical school at one of the eight regional campuses, while one-third of medical students begin medical school in Indianapolis. For decades, and in contrast to most other states, the Indiana system delivered the first two years of medical education distributed among nine cities, followed by clinical rotations converging at Indianapolis. From 2006 to 2016, concomitant with the overall expansion of the IU School of Medicine, the regional campuses systematically expanded from first and second year campuses to four-year campuses capable of educating medical students in the first through fourth years. As the popularity of university "towns" has grown for youth, families, alumni, and retiring baby-boomers, the regional medical campus at Bloomington became the largest outside of Indianapolis. Bloomington can be reached from Indianapolis in less than 90 minutes via a new interstate highway, reflecting Indiana's prominence as an international supply chain and transportation center for the enormous medical device and pharmaceutical distribution industries.

At Bloomington, the medical sciences faculty of the regional medical campus teaches throughout the collegiate, graduate, and medical degree programs. Whereas Indiana University supports two schools of law and two schools of public health, the Indiana University School of Medicine's nine-campus system operates as one medical school and teaches one statewide curriculum. As one multi-campus school of medicine, the IU School of Medicine has earned its full reaccreditation consistently, most recently in 2017 through 2025.

Structure, Governance and Funding:

Indiana University is governed by its Board of Trustees, including, in recent years, two IU medical students who serve in successive terms. At Bloomington, the Provost is the chief academic officer. From Indianapolis, the Dean of IU School of Medicine also serves as the Executive Vice President for University Clinical Affairs. IU medical students lead the extensive statewide medical student council, student interest groups, peer-mentoring programs, and serve on statewide curriculum committees and subcommittees.

Student Body:

Statewide, 83 percent (n = 302 of 364) of IU medical students originate from in-state. Similarly, at Bloomington, 78 percent (n = 28 of 36) of medical students are in-state. For the 2018-2019 academic year, the plan for the number of first, second, third, and fourth medical students at the Bloomington regional campus is the following:

Number of students per academic year 2018-2019

> First year = 39
> Second year = 32
> Third year = 8
> Fourth year = 8

One Admissions Committee is responsible for all offers of admission to the IU School of Medicine. Offers occur on a rolling basis periodically throughout the interview season. A preference ranking system leads to the initial assignment to a campus location. A campus assignment committee reviews special requests for campus re-assignments. Using online, webinar, and in-person resources, students applying to IU School of Medicine learn of the unique statewide system of medical education.

Match results of medical students completing the longitudinal integrated curriculum (LIC), offered only at Bloomington, demonstrate a 100 percent match rate. The overall school match rate reflects the national match rate of 95 percent. Twenty-eight students have completed the third year Bloomington LIC ("BLIC") since its inception in 2012. Twenty-four students (86 percent) have matched in the following disciplines: Emergency Medicine, Family Medicine, Internal Medicine, OB-GYN, Pediatrics, Psychiatry, and Surgery. Four students (14 percent) matched in Anesthesia, Dermatology, and Radiology. The prevalence of community-hospital disciplines and primary care career paths reflects the experience and competence students gain from their education by outstanding medical staff at the 273-bed IU Health Bloomington Hospital, along with affiliated hospitals in adjacent rural counties.. Students work one-to-one with attending physicians, many of whom are alumni of IU and IU School of Medicine.

Curriculum:

The regional medical campus at Bloomington, the largest outside Indianapolis, offers the only longitudinal clinical clerkship spanning the clerkship year in Indiana. The Bloomington LIC fulfills the requirements of the statewide medical curriculum, although arranged and delivered differently. Clinical experiences vary in duration from two weeks, a semester, and a year to optimize the educational experiences for the medical students, individually and in small groups. Challenges include recruitment and retention of sufficient clinical preceptors in the specialties of Neurology, OB-GYN, and Psychiatry, mostly reflecting uneven distribution statewide.

Unique Characteristics:

The majority of regional medical students at Bloomington take advantage of research and clinical opportunities: regional, national, and international. These opportunities are supported by stipends and scholarships totaling in excess of $100,000 annually and culminating in poster presentations regionally and statewide.

Campus strengths also include the education track of the Ph.D. program in Anatomy, as well as doctoral and graduate programs, including

Cell, Molecular, and Cancer Biology. University strengths include the following: IU Kelley School of Business; IU School of Music; and educational expertise in world languages, along with a vast array of degree programs, majors, and institutes offered at the picturesque Hoosier campus of Indiana University.

Accomplishments and Challenges:

The integrated longitudinal curriculum, the extensive resources for student research and clinical experiences, and the 100 percent match rate are three standout features of the regional medical campus at Bloomington. A challenge for the regional campus would be to elevate the brand visibility of the internationally recognized IU School of Medicine in and around the university campus.

Future Plans:

In 2021, a new Regional Academic Health Center (RAHC) will replace the current hospital, serving Bloomington and south central Indiana. As part of the overall $400 million dollar investment, a new academic building will feature instructional space for inter-professional education, a new simulation center, and new academic homes for speech and hearing, nursing, social work, and medicine.

4. Medical College of Georgia, Southeast Regional Campus

Authors:

- Turner W. Rentz, Jr., M.D.,
  Associate Dean SE Regional Campus,
  Associate Professor of Surgery,
  Medical College of Georgia

- Frances Purcell, Ph.D.,
  Assistant Dean for Curriculum, SE Regional Campus,
  Assistant Professor of Psychiatry and Health Behavior,
  Medical College of Georgia

Regional Campus:

Medical College of Georgia, Southeast Regional Campus
Location: Savannah and Brunswick, Georgia

Institution (main campus):

Medical College of Georgia at Augusta University
Location: Augusta, Georgia

History and Mission:

The Medical College of Georgia, a unit of the University System of Georgia, was founded in 1828 and is the only public medical school in Georgia. Its mission is to train physicians for the state, provide tertiary care for its citizens and to support medical research. Over 50 percent of the physicians in Georgia either trained or attended medical school at MCG.

In response to a growing national recognition of an impending physician shortage, the governor of Georgia tasked the medical schools to increase their enrollment. The state of Georgia had one-third as many physicians, residents in training, and medical students as Michigan, a state with a comparable population. Funding to support Regional Medical Campus expansion was provided by the legislature as an embedded line item in the state budget, which persists today. As the state's public medical school, the Medical College of Georgia embraced the goal of expansion. The Medical College of Georgia, with the support of the Board of Regents, decided to develop regional clinical campuses rather than building a second medical school. The goals of the regional concept were to not only increase the number of physicians, but to encourage a more even distribution of healthcare professionals by educating them in community hospitals in rural and urban areas.

The first of the regional campuses was the Southwest campus in Albany, which started in 2006. In 2010, the Southeast campus was the second of three regional campuses to be developed and began at the same time that our partnership four-year campus in Athens, Georgia was started. The Northwest campus in Rome, Georgia, was started in 2013.

Our first Southeast campus dean, Dr. Kathryn Martin, was hired in 2008 to help get the campus up and running. As she was walking across the campus in Augusta, one of the first-year students approached her and said he wanted to be on the Southeast campus. She told him that we didn't have a campus yet, to which he said, "yes, but you will". He was one of the original seven students who did most of their third year on the Southeast campus as a pilot program in 2010. In 2011 we were approved for 20 students for their third and fourth years. We now have

20 third, 20 fourth, and 10 to 20 rotating students from the main campus each month. Our clinical faculty, who are all unpaid volunteers, now number over 300.

Our clinical campus is unusual with two main hospital systems: one based in Brunswick, Georgia at Southeast Georgia Health System and the other in Savannah, Georgia at Saint Joseph's/Candler Health System, which have a combined bed capacity of over 1,000 inpatient beds. Both have administrative suites that were donated to the campuses by their hospital systems and are located 190 and 125 miles from the main campus, respectively. Brunswick and Savannah are 85 miles apart and our students complete the majority of their courses at one or the other campus, with the rest of their courses occurring at other sites in the Southeast region. Clerkships are taught at both sites that comprise the Southeast Regional Campus, and all students spend time in both locations.

Structure, Governance and Funding:

The Southeast Regional Campus was started with one Associate Dean and soon added an Assistant Dean for Curriculum. The Associate Dean reports to an Associate Dean for Regional Campuses who provides a unified voice to the Senior Associate Dean for Undergraduate Medical Education at the main campus.

Funding for regional campus expansion is provided by the legislature as an imbedded line item in the state budget and is administered by the Associate Dean for Regional Campuses and the Senior Associate Dean for Undergraduate Medical Education of the school.

The campus suites in Savannah and Brunswick are provided by the hospitals at no cost. Both suites have full AV and teleconference connections to the main campus. The regional deans are members of the governing committees of the main campus and meet in person with other deans and chairs at the monthly Deans Staff Meeting. There are also monthly meetings for the regional deans, as well as participation on the Curriculum Oversight Committee, Promotions Committee, and Admission Committee.

Student Body:

The student body of the southeast campus mirrors that of the main campus of the Medical College of Georgia. Over 90 percent are in-state students and are an ethnically diverse group, which represents the population of Georgia. In order to recruit students to the regional campuses, the regional campus deans travel to Augusta each fall and present the details of each regional campus.

Students apply to the regional campus in the fall of their second year and are selected by an Admissions Committee consisting of students, clinical faculty, and campus leadership. Applicants are usually notified of their acceptance by Thanksgiving.

Each of the regional deans then meet with the new students early in the next year to introduce them to the campus and help with student clerkship selection.

Our student's specialty selection on the regional campus is identical to that of the main campus. About 50 percent of our students choose primary care specialties, and the others are divided among the other specialties at about the same percentages as the main campus.

Curriculum:

The Southeast Regional Campus curriculum models the curriculum offered on the main campus during the third and fourth years. Students in their core curriculum are connected to the main campus for academic half days and participate in many activities on the main campus. Regional campus Site Directors report to a Clerkship Director on the main campus, and likewise, Regional Coordinators work with Clerkship Coordinators on the main campus for administrative support. Most clerkship assignments are made through the lottery system on the main campus, but the regional campus can assign electives and certain clerkships. All changes to the curriculum are governed by the Curriculum Oversight Committee to ensure adherence to the school's competency-based objectives. The regional deans write the Medical Student Performance Evaluations (MSPE) for Southeast Regional Campus students.

Unique Characteristics:

The Southeast campus is unique with two main supporting hospitals and two campus suites. The Assistant Dean for Curriculum is housed in Savannah and the campus Associate Dean has his main office in Brunswick with administrative suites in both hospital systems. Our campus is large and covers 35 counties in Southeast Georgia, which provides both opportunities and challenges.

Accomplishments and Challenges:

Our students have done well. Their grades, Step and NBME scores have been equal to or better than those on the main campus and nationally.

Since the first group in 2010, our students have matched well, and many are now completing their postgraduate training.

We, like other regional campuses, face challenges with preceptor and site development. As a state institution, we cannot pay faculty, but we compete with other schools that do. We also compete with other health professional students for teaching sites throughout the state. We rely on the loyalty of alumni, and the desire of professionals to help educate the next generation of physicians. Additional challenges include the development of regional clinical research opportunities, housing, and clinical faculty education. As preceptor growth allows, we would like to eventually increase enrollment to 30 third- and fourth-year students.

5. Medical College of Wisconsin-Central Wisconsin

Authors:

- Lisa Grill Dodson, M.D.,
  Campus Dean,
  Professor of Family and Community Medicine,
  Medical College of Wisconsin- Central Wisconsin

- Courtney Schwebach MS II,
  Medical College of Wisconsin-Central Wisconsin

Regional Campus:

Medical College of Wisconsin-Central Wisconsin
Location: Wausau, Wisconsin

Institution (main campus):

Medical College of Wisconsin
Location: Milwaukee, Wisconsin

History and Mission:

Founded in 1893, the Medical College of Wisconsin (MCW) celebrates its 125th year in Milwaukee in 2018. The focus throughout its history has been the greater Milwaukee area. With the call by the AAMC and others for class size expansion to address projected physician shortages, and the arrival of a new president, John R. Raymond, Sr., M.D. and

Dean, Joseph E. Kerschner, M.D., MCW began exploration of expansion into areas of the state previously underutilized for medical education. The intention was targeted and mission-driven class size expansion through regional campuses, with a specific mission to address workforce shortages in northern Wisconsin, particularly in primary care and psychiatry. MCW-Central Wisconsin (MCW-CW) in Wausau, WI is one of two regional campuses of MCW, with the other located in Green Bay. The regional campuses were established and accredited in 2016 (CW) and 2015 (GB). The Central Wisconsin campus is 180 miles northeast of Milwaukee, and 100 miles west of Green Bay.

Structure, Governance, and Funding:

MCW-CW is a regional campus of MCW-Milwaukee. The campus is led by a Campus Dean who reports directly to the Dean and Provost of the School of Medicine. An Assistant Dean for Basic Sciences, an Assistant Dean for Clinical Learning, and a Campus Administrator report to the Campus Dean. This team works closely with Milwaukee-based Academic Affairs leadership to plan and implement curriculum, provide student services and ensure comparability between campuses. The regional campus faculty consists of both basic science and clinical faculty who monitor students in the basic science courses, provide tutoring and connection to the main campus departments, offer campus-based advising, and conduct small group learning. In addition, local physicians serve as small group leaders, content experts, mentors, and clinical teachers. Students and faculty have representation on key MCW committees, including Curriculum and Evaluation, Academic Standing, Student Assembly, and Faculty Council. In addition, they are also involved in individual course planning, assessment committees, and student organization leadership positions.

Student Body:

The MCW regional campuses in Central Wisconsin and Green Bay developed a highly community-engaged admissions process, utilizing a Regional Admissions Advisory Committee (RAAC). The RAAC consists of approximately 30 community leaders from relevant stakeholder groups, including physicians and other medical providers, faculty, business, philanthropy, education, patient advocacy, community development, and faith communities. The regional campus dean selects RAAC volunteers who are then jointly trained by the regional campus and MCW admissions committee. Application to MCW is through AMCAS. The MCW Admissions Committee initially screens all applicants for academic standards. Successfully screened candidates receive a secondary application, and may then indicate a campus preference. Applicants who rank a regional campus are then screened for specific campus fit by at least two RAAC members at the appropriate campus. Half-day, campus-specific interviews are conducted on the regional campuses, and include a 30-minute panel interview by six to eight RAAC and one or two MCW Admissions Committee members. Admissions recommendations are made for each applicant, and sent to the MCW Admissions Committee for review and approval. Admissions decisions are made on a rolling basis. Accepted students tend toward Wisconsin residents (87 percent), with a primary care or psychiatry career interest, and rural or small-town experience. Applicants with medicine as a second career, geographic, economic, and ethnic diversity, and other life experiences are encouraged.

Curriculum:

The MCW regional campuses in Central Wisconsin and Green Bay offer a year-round curriculum, allowing completion of all MCW graduation requirements in three calendar years. Twenty-five students are admitted directly to the campus and complete their full medical school experience on the regional campus. Therefore, students can expect to complete their education in three years, but may extend to a four-year experience. Approximately 70 percent of students are anticipated to complete the curriculum in three years. The campuses are highly connected, and didactic lectures and other large group activities are delivered simultaneously to all campuses by two-way audio visual technology. In addition, all didactic sessions are recorded and live streamed. Small group (team and problem based) learning and laboratories are conducted in groups of six to eight students.

The accelerated curriculum is accomplished by starting earlier and going year-round. Students have standard winter and spring breaks, but begin clinical work full-time during the summer between M1 (first) and M2 (second) year through the Central Wisconsin Integrated Clerkship (CWIC), our version of a Longitudinal Integrated Clerkship (LIC). Due to the accelerated nature of the three-year curriculum, some curricular elements are reordered. For example, Foundations of Clinical Medicine, the basic doctoring course, is taught as a five-week summer block prior to the matriculation of the four-year students in Milwaukee. Regional campus students are then prepared to enter Clinical Apprenticeship, a half-day per week clinical experience, a semester earlier. Other elements of the traditional M2 year, including OSCE assessments, are moved into the M1 year, preparing students to undertake clinical work during CWIC. Students return to systems-based M2 Pathophysiology courses, taken simultaneously with students from all campuses. Additional advanced clinical instruction and assessment is completed during the M2 year, and students return to CWIC in the summer between the M2 and M3 year.

All MCW students participate in an individualized learning project through completion of the Scholarly Pathways Program. The sole MCW-CW Scholarly Pathway is "Physician in the Community". Through this pathway, students are introduced to community leaders and agencies working in areas related to social determinants of health. The students then work with a community and faculty mentor to create a service project that addresses a community need. The pathway combines service learning, research, and the community to teach students how to be agents of change in a meaningful and productive way. In addition, students learn the importance of ethics in research as IRB approval is sought for all projects.

Students may "decelerate" or extend to a four-year curriculum at several points, for personal, academic, or career choice reasons. The determination for the deceleration varies based on the underlying factors, but requires the recommendation of the Campus Dean and approval of the Associate Dean of Student Affairs.

Unique Characteristics:

The small class size (25 per year) offers students a leadership role in shaping the campus and curriculum. Utilization of a three-year community engaged curriculum, Longitudinal Integrated Clerkship (LIC) model, and individualized scholarly work on a regional campus make the MCW-Central Wisconsin campus unique in the US. Attending physicians and residents frequently teach on a one-on-one basis, providing individualized learning opportunities and mentoring. Students establish meaningful continuity relationships with communities, teaching physicians, and patients.

Accomplishment and Challenges:

Students on all MCW campuses exhibit comparable academic performance. Achieving acceptance and understanding by residencies, accreditors, and others for a three-year competency-based, rather than time-based, curriculum remains a challenge, despite an increasing national dialogue around competency-based curriculum reform. Limited student interest in primary care is a national concern that can only partially be mitigated with local attention to admissions and curriculum.

Future Plans:

We will be monitoring the long-term effect of placing a medical school campus in a rural community, and community health outcomes related to student Scholarly Pathway projects completed with community agencies.

6. Mercer University School of Medicine, Columbus Campus

Authors:

- Alice Aumann House, M.D.
  Regional Dean, Columbus Campus,
  Senior Associate Dean of Admissions and Student Affairs,
  Professor of Family Medicine,
  Mercer University School of Medicine, Columbus Campus

- Chris Scoggins, MPH,
  Director, Mercer Community Preceptor Network,
  Assistant Director,
  Community Outreach and Population Health,
  Instructor, Department of Community Medicine,
  Mercer University School of Medicine, Columbus Campus

Regional Campus:

Mercer University School of Medicine, Columbus Campus
Location: Columbus, Georgia

Institution (main campus):

Mercer University School of Medicine
Location: Macon, Georgia

History and Mission:

Since our inception in 1982, the mission of Mercer University's School of Medicine (SOM) in Macon, Georgia has been to educate physicians for rural, underserved areas of the state. While as early as the 1990s, Mercer University began educating clinical students in Columbus, Georgia in the third-year family medicine rotation, the school also formally expanded to include an additional four-year campus in Savannah in 2008. The regional campus in Columbus is geographically suited to anchor efforts in the most underserved, impoverished, and rural areas of the state.

The new Columbus regional medical campus (RMC) was designed to:

1. Train third- and fourth-year Mercer University medical students after two years at the Macon or Savannah campus.

2. Address shortages in primary care and health care disparities in rural Georgia.

3. Facilitate a collaborative relationship between two hospital systems in Columbus — Columbus Regional Midtown Medical Center and St. Francis Hospital.

The first full-time Senior Associate Dean of the campus was selected to oversee expansion of clinical opportunities, provide oversight for the clinical faculty, and foster relationships between the teaching hospitals and the medical school. The first group of students volunteered to transfer to Columbus in 2012. The campus has subsequently expanded in class size, growing from 15 to 20 students per class year. The first class graduated in 2014. The Columbus campus is located on the western border of the state with the main campus in Macon, in the middle of the state, and the Savannah Campus on the eastern edge of the state.

Structure, Governance, and Funding:

During our first year, the campus was overseen by a part-time campus dean, who split time between the main campus and the Columbus campus. This quickly transitioned to a full-time Senior Associate Dean who reports directly to the Dean of the School of Medicine. In addition, an Assistant Dean of Clinical Education has been appointed at each of the two teaching hospitals. The Senior Associate Dean collaborates closely with leadership in Academic Affairs, Student Affairs, and Faculty Affairs, some of whom are located on other campuses.

Funding comes primarily from the state legislature through the main campus budget. Such funding has helped us to expand from a single office and classroom (donated by one of the teaching hospitals), to a suite of offices and classrooms with video-conferencing capabilities in a historic building located in uptown Columbus.

Student Body:

Pursuant to the school's mission, all students are Georgia residents. Preference is given to students from rural areas with strong ties to the state. The school accepts 120 students per class with 60 students on each of the Macon and Savannah campuses for the pre-clinical years. The first four classes in Columbus volunteered to attend the regional campus during their second year. Students now choose the Columbus campus at the time of matriculation. The Columbus campus accepts up to 20 students in both the third- and fourth-year classes. Columbus students are comparable to the greater student body in most metrics, and therefore, no selection bias is evident. Students can complete all of their clinical experiences on the Columbus campus. To date, more than 80 percent of Columbus campus graduates have selected core specialties for residency

(Family Medicine, Internal Medicine, Pediatrics, General Surgery, OB GYN, or Emergency Medicine).

Curriculum:

The Columbus curriculum mirrors the curriculum at the Macon and the Savannah campuses. There are six core third-year clerkships (Family Medicine, Internal Medicine, OB GYN, Pediatrics, Psychiatry, and General Surgery), overseen by clerkship directors equally distributed between the two teaching hospitals. Clinical rotations are distributed equally between the two teaching hospitals and students receive a great deal of one-on-one instruction from faculty including hands-on training in the operating and delivery rooms. The fourth-year curriculum also mirrors that of the other campuses by offering a wide variety of required and elective courses. Students participate in a longitudinal Radiology and Healthcare Topics course via video-conferencing to one of the other campuses. The Senior Capstone course and graduation are on the main campus. Mercer offers an accelerated track in Family Medicine for students wishing to complete their degree in three years with a guaranteed seat in the Columbus Regional Family Medicine Residency program. The MSPE is written by the Senior Associate Dean for Admissions and Student Affairs on the Columbus campus.

Unique Characteristics:

In general, Mercer University SOM offers small class sizes and a clinical faculty that works closely with the students. The Columbus campus offers a smaller class size and more direct contact with faculty. With the classroom and administrative offices being located on the river front in historic uptown Columbus, the students have access to a vibrant and active social life.

Our students are active in the community and have started several service opportunities that benefit the underserved populations in the community including an organization to provide opportunities for special needs children to participate in 5k and half marathon races.

All of our students receive a primary care clinical advisor upon arriving at the Columbus campus that helps them navigate the complexities of the clinical rotations and residency selection.

Accomplishments and Challenges:

Over 80 percent of Columbus campus students select a core specialty for their residency training. Despite a short history, several graduates have already returned to practice locally and meet the mission of the school.

As is true on all Mercer campuses, recruiting, training, and supporting a voluntary clinical faculty is the greatest challenge. With an unopposed Family Medicine residency as the only graduate medical program, the Columbus campus is more dependent on volunteer clinical faculty than sites with multiple residency programs. Faculty development is a challenge due to the busy clinical schedules and the lack of protected time for such activities. To provide faculty development, the faculty affairs dean travels to the campus periodically and sessions are available by video-conferencing. The student financial planning staff from the main campus visits the campus regularly and the campus dean acts as the primary point of contact for most of the other student services.

Future Plans:

It is Mercer's goal to develop a four-year campus with a focus on clinical research in Columbus, Georgia. The campus would provide a comparable curriculum and experience to the other campuses across all four years of the curriculum. All development plans are in close collaboration with community stakeholders and (to the greatest extent possible), aligned with local development objectives. An increased medical education infrastructure supports development of the medical community in Columbus and has been embraced by the local hospitals, city government, and chamber of commerce.

7. Northern Medical Program, University of British Columbia

Authors:

- Sean B. Maurice, Ph.D.,
  Senior Lab Instructor, *University of Northern British Columbia;*
  Foundations of Medical Practice Site Director, *Northern Medical Program, University of British Columbia*

- Paul J. Winwood, MB, BS, DM, FRCPC,
  Regional Associate Dean, Northern British Columbia,
  University of British Columbia;
  Associate Vice President, *Northern Medical Program, University of Northern British Columbia*

Regional Campus:

Northern Medical Program, University of British Columbia
Location: University of Northern British Columbia,
Prince George, British Columbia

Institution (main campus):

University of British Columbia MD Undergraduate Program
Location: Vancouver, British Columbia

History and Mission:

In the late 1990s, the province of British Columbia (BC) was facing a significant physician shortage, with far fewer new physicians graduating each year than needed and an aging physician demographic. This shortage was felt most severely in northern and rural regions of the province where physician recruitment and retention had always been difficult.

The resource-intensive town of Prince George (population ~ 85,000) is the healthcare hub of North Central BC, serving a population of 350,000 people spread across a vast geography, comparable to the size of France. In 2000, physician shortages in Prince George reached a breaking point. A rally was held, attended by over 7,000 community members, after which local leaders proposed the creation of a medical school in Prince George. This was approved by the provincial government and, in January 2001, a memorandum of agreement was signed between the University of Northern British Columbia (UNBC) and the University of British Columbia (UBC) to develop a Regional Medical Campus (RMC), the Northern Medical Program (NMP), of the University of British Columbia MD Undergraduate Program (MDUP) at UNBC.

In 2004, 24 students started in the NMP which was part of a province-wide expansion of the MDUP. In 2011, the intake increased to 32 students per year[1]. The main goal of the NMP was to train physicians for northern, rural, and regional practice. Other goals included: training with a primary care and generalist perspective, a focus on working in indigenous communities, access to medical education for students from northern and rural BC, and improvement in healthcare services in northern BC.

Structure, Governance and Funding:

The UBC MDUP is delivered in partnership with UNBC with whom there is an affiliation agreement describing governance, the academic program, students, faculty, funding, and facilities. Students receive their M.D. degrees from UBC.

The Dean of the UBC Faculty of Medicine is administratively responsible for the conduct and quality of the NMP, acting through a Regional Associate Dean (RAD) who reports to the Dean, the Executive Associate Dean for Education, UBC, and the Provost of UNBC. The RAD is supported by an Assistant Dean and local Site Course Directors, who coordinate with Course Directors at other sites, in addition to local faculty and an administrative team.

Provincial funding and tuition fees for the NMP flow through both UBC and UNBC. Funds are held and administered at UNBC. The Distributed Program Planning Committee, a group with representation from UBC and the partner institutions, approves the annual budget and allocation of resources and recommends it to the Dean.

Student Body:

All students in the MDUP complete their first semester of medical school together at the main campus, and then students in the NMP move to the regional campus in Prince George for the start of the winter semester.

Admission to the program is handled through the main campus and applicants apply concomitantly for all sites, ranking their location of choice. A Rural and Remote Suitability Score tool is used to place appropriate value on the strengths of rural and remote applicants. It includes an assessment of rural background, community ties, and experiences and activities in a rural setting. This is mandatory for all applicants to the NMP[2]. A Northern and Rural Admissions Selection Committee adjudicates the applications.

An Assistant Dean of Student Affairs is available to support students at the RMC, and reports to the Associate Dean of Student Affairs at the main UBC campus.

Curriculum:

At the initial distribution, years one and two of the UBC MDUP moved to a Problem-Based Learning Curriculum (PBL), supplemented by video-conferenced lectures, with the majority being broadcast from the main campus. Dedicated bandwidth and technicians at all sites ensure greater than 99.5 percent reliability of the synchronous video-conferencing. Small group sessions are delivered at the regional campus using local faculty. From the first semester, students start clinical skills training and family practice office visits.

Laboratories are delivered synchronously across sites. A virtual histology platform with high resolution digital images is accessible to the entire class concurrently[3,4]. For gross anatomy, cadaver dissection occurs at all sites.

Students across all UBC sites participate in a rural family practice rotation in the third year to provide exposure to rural family medicine. During clerkships, all the major specialties are taught at the NMP. While some subspecialty areas are not available in Northern BC, students can experience any area of medicine during year four, which consists of province-wide electives and up to eight weeks out of province. Two very successful Longitudinal Integrated Clerkship (LIC) Programs were created at affiliated medical centers in smaller towns within our region (population ~20,000). Eight students per year complete their clerkship in an LIC format.

Since 2015, UBC has introduced a renewed curriculum with an integrated spiral and developmental structure. It is competency based with programmatic assessment and focuses on clinical decision making, with longitudinal themes underpinned by principles of social accountability, excellence, professionalism, scholarship, diversity, and equity. Case-based Learning has replaced PBL and transitional courses into clinical experiences and practice (i.e. residency) have been introduced. Foundations of Scholarship and Flexible Enhanced Learning courses have been added which give students the opportunity to explore their own lines of scholarly inquiry. The program was accredited in 2008 and 2016, and, in both cases accreditors determined that the pre-clinical and clinical training across all sites of the MDUP was comparable.

Unique Characteristics:

The vast geography in which NMP students learn provides an immersive experience in rural healthcare. The community of Prince George, and other communities across Northern BC, has been hugely supportive of the local university and the NMP. This is evidenced by the formation of the Northern Medical Programs Trust, to which 29 communities and local governments donate annually to support students learning in the north. The community is incredibly proud of the NMP and students encounter this daily when seeing patients.

The NMP is in the smallest city of any site in the MDUP, with the lowest number of practicing physicians per medical student. This means that the program requires and has very significant engagement from the physician community, with more than 90 percent of local physicians involved in teaching. The students benefit from a large amount of hands-on time, broad clinical exposure, and low student to faculty ratios (often 1:1) in the clinical years.

Accomplishments and Challenges:

Graduates from the NMP have been highly successful in obtaining residencies of their choosing anywhere across the country in every specialty, (with more than 90 percent in their first choice discipline and more than 96 percent in the first round CaRMS match). Overall, 58 percent of NMP graduates have entered family practice and 67 percent of those in independent practice are working in rural and northern BC.

Maintaining physician engagement and fostering a teaching culture is essential for the NMP and is a priority area. Understanding and addressing the barriers to teaching is an ongoing challenge.

Future Plans:

The NMP is transitioning from the initial establishment phase to growing and sustaining the program into the future. We are building our research programs alongside our education programs with a Northern and rural focus. To help ensure a pipeline of future physicians for Northern and rural BC, we are focusing on community engagement, including a program to support socioeconomically disadvantaged undergraduate students in Northern BC who aspire to enter medical school.

References:

1. Faculty of Medicine Education, University of British Columbia (December 6, 2013). Faculty of Medicine Education Infographic. Retrieved June 22, 2017 from http://www.med. ubc.ca/faculty-of-medicine-education-infographic/

2. Bates, J., Casiro, O., Fleming, B., Frinton, V., Towle, A., & Snadden, D. (2005). Expanding undergraduate medical education in British Columbia: a distributed campus model. Canadian Medical Education Journal. 173(6), 1-7.

3. Pinder, K. E., Ford, J. C., & Ovalle, W. K. (2008). A New Paradigm for Teaching Histology Laboratories in Canada's First Distributed Medical School. Anatomical Sciences Education. 1(3): 95-101.

4. Department of Cellular & Physiological Sciences, University of British Columbia (2004). Virtual Histology. Retrieved June 27, 2017 from http://cps.med.ubc.ca/virtual-histology/

8. Penn State College of Medicine, University Park Campus

Authors:

- E. Eugene Marsh, M.D.,
  Founding Senior Associate Dean for Education,
  Professor of Neurology and Master Educator,
  Penn State College of Medicine, University Park Campus

- Michael P. Flanagan, M.D., FAAFP
  Assistant Dean for Student Affairs,
  Professor and Vice-Chair of Family and Community Medicine,
  Penn State College of Medicine, University Park Campus

Regional Campus:

Penn State College of Medicine, University Park Program
Location: State College, Pennsylvania

Institution (main campus):

Penn State College of Medicine, Hershey Program
Location: Hershey, Pennsylvania

History and Mission:

In 1965, the Penn State College of Medicine was founded in Hershey, Pennsylvania, 100 miles south of Penn State University. In 2010 a decision was made to develop a Regional Medical Campus in State College,

Pennsylvania, adjacent to the University's main campus. The *University Park (UP) Regional Campus* was launched the following year.

The primary goals for the new regional campus were to:

(1) Facilitate partnerships between the Penn State College of Medicine (PSCOM) and the Hershey Medical Center, such as research, interprofessional training, and dual degree programs.
(2) Address the primary care shortage and health disparities in rural Pennsylvania.
(3) Enhance clinical services for the State College community.
(4) Train third- and fourth-year Penn State medical students, after two years of training at the Hershey campus.

A Professor of Neurology and Senior Associate Dean from the University of Alabama Tuscaloosa was recruited as the inaugural Senior Associate Dean for the new campus. Arriving in 2011, he helped to expand the existing clinical presence in State College. Seventeen years prior to this, the Penn State Orthopaedic Surgery and Sports Medicine Group was established to care for Penn State athletes, and the Penn State Family Medicine group was founded to provide primary care for the University's faculty and staff. This small group of faculty hosted one to two medical students each month when the regional campus was created. However, there were few other PSCOM faculty present during this time.

Like most regional campuses, we were highly dependent on community physicians and the local medical center to build the educational infrastructure. With a supportive and forward-thinking community hospital CEO and board, we successfully engaged the large physician group employed by the hospital as potential clinical teaching faculty. LCME

(Liaison Committee on Medical Education) consultation was obtained in August of 2011, with subsequent accreditation.

The first group of students was recruited from the second year class in Hershey. These 13 "pioneers" who started their third year of training in 2012 at the UP Campus, proved critical to our building efforts, and helped us continue to create relationships within the community for subsequent classes. This original cohort graduated in 2014, uniformly matching into their preferred residency programs.

Structure, Governance and Funding:

While we started with one Senior Associate Dean at the UP campus, this transitioned to a UP Vice-Dean who answered directly to the College of Medicine Dean, and an Associate Dean for Education who reported to both the UP Vice-Dean and the Vice-Dean for Education at the main campus. An Assistant Dean for Student Affairs was subsequently added to prepare for a four-year campus.

Our primary source of funding in the early years was the main campus of Penn State University and the local independent medical center. Eventually, a local state senator was successful in establishing a state grant for the regional campus. This grant, along with matching federal funds, allowed us to expand our educational infrastructure, assist with student housing costs, establish a Student Learning Center, and develop curricular innovations as we planned for expansion to a four-year medical campus.

Student Body:

The University Park Regional Campus began with 13 third-year students recruited from the second-year class at the main campus in Hershey. Most of their clinical training occurred in State College at the regional medical center and local outpatient offices. Major events, such as graduation and white-coat ceremony, still occurred at the main campus in Hershey with the entire class.

Graduates from the regional campus have been highly successful in the "Match", with students moving on to training programs at Yale, Johns Hopkins, and Harvard, among others. Although students at our University Park Campus can choose any specialty, to date approximately 42 percent of our graduates have pursued primary care careers.

Curriculum:

The UP curriculum originally reflected the main campus curriculum. Initially, these were in traditional block rotations coordinated by local clerkship directors. Ultimate oversight was provided by the clerkship directors in Hershey, but was transitioned to the UP clerkship directors after two years. The regional campus deans generate Medical Student Performance Evaluations (MSPE) for UP students in preparation for residency interviews.

Since 2015, four students per year participated in a complete longitudinal integrated clerkship (LIC). By 2016, all of our students participated in a Family and Community Medicine LIC. Subsequently, in 2017, LICs were in place for all UP students in Family Medicine, Internal Medicine, Pediatrics, OB/GYN, and Surgery. The positive experience of the Clerkship Directors with the LIC cohort facilitated the expansion of the longitudinal approach, with all core clerkships being delivered as an LIC in 2018.

Unique Characteristics:

Compared to the main campus in Hershey, the UP campus offers smaller class sizes, more direct contact with teaching faculty, and a community focus that may foster an interest in primary care and/or practice in underserved areas. Living in a college town is attractive to students because of a wide range of extracurricular options. Dual degree programs were an original goal of the regional campus. The first approved dual degree, an M.D./ MBA program, took advantage of the adjacent Penn State College of Business. M.D. /Ph.D. programs are also available, and M.D./ MPH dual degrees soon followed.

Our third-year students have created opportunities that are comparable to those at the main campus. They established a student-run free clinic, LionCare, within four years of launching the regional campus, modeled after a similar student-run clinic near Hershey. All Penn State College of Medicine students must complete a Medical Student Research Project (MSRP) and proximity to the main campus has facilitated collaboration.

Career and academic advising for our students was initially approached by honoring advising relationships established at the Hershey Campus in the pre-clinical years, while concurrently matching each student with one local faculty advisor in the specialty of their choice. Because two-thirds of our UP teaching faculty are employed by the local medical center and not the PSCOM, many career advisors were community-based physicians with a clinical teaching appointment. With expansion to a four-year campus, career and academic advising was provided at the University Park campus by the Assistant Dean for Student Affairs. In addition, each student is matched with a specific specialty advisor at the main academic medical campus during their third year.

Accomplishments and Challenges:

Like many regional campuses, the Penn State College of Medicine University Park Campus represents an ideal venue for innovation in medical education. Most recently, we have developed a four-year curriculum that will nearly eliminate lectures in favor of small group tutorial sessions, and incorporate clinical, as well as basic science experiences throughout the curriculum from the very beginning. For example, first year medical students are immersed in primary care clinics soon after matriculation, and then draw on this experience to facilitate case-based learning. Other accomplishments include establishing novel Medical Humanities selectives, an innovative retreat to promote resilience and moving the clerkship rotations to the second year.

Recruiting, training, and maintaining a voluntary physician workforce probably represents the greatest challenge for our campus going forward. Other challenges that require careful attention include maintaining comparability with the main campus, as required by the LCME, and ensuring the same level of student academic support and remediation. As we move to a four-year campus, our challenges are primarily related to developing an innovative curriculum with the same level of student services and extracurricular opportunities that exist at the Hershey campus. Finally, as the regional campus activities grow at a rate that sometimes seems exponential, ensuring that we have adequate staffing of both faculty and administrative support is paramount.

Future Plans:

Developing a full-service, four-year campus at University Park with an innovative curriculum that incorporates clinical experiences from the start, and providing the faculty and administrative support required to accomplish this, is our current focus. Involving medical students in designing this new curriculum is part of our creative innovation.

9. Temple/St. Luke's School of Medicine

Authors:

- Joel C. Rosenfeld, M.D., M.Ed.,
  Chief Academic Officer,
  St. Luke's University Health Network,
  Senior Associate Dean and Professor of Surgery,
  Lewis Katz School of Medicine at Temple University

- Kathleen A. Dave, Ph.D.,
  Assistant Dean for Student Affairs,
  Clinical Assistant Professor of Neurology,
  Lewis Katz School of Medicine at Temple University/
  St. Luke's University Health Network

Regional Campus:

Temple/St. Luke's School of Medicine
Location: Bethlehem, Pennsylvania

Institution (main campus):

Lewis Katz School of Medicine at Temple University
Location: Philadelphia, Pennsylvania

History and Mission:

For more than 50 years, St. Luke's University Health Network (SLUHN) has been involved in medical student education. Initially, students from Temple University School of Medicine (TUSM) came to St. Luke's for some of their clinical rotations. In 2006, TUSM and St. Luke's established a clinical campus for 16 third-year and 16 fourth-year students at St. Luke's University Hospital in Bethlehem, PA, approximately 60 miles north of TUSM. These students completed all required clinical rotations and most of their electives at St. Luke's. Realizing that there was going to be a significant physician shortage, St. Luke's wanted to train more future physicians. This led to the founding of the Temple University School of Medicine/St. Luke's University Health Network Regional Medical School campus (Temple/St. Luke's) in 2011. TUSM then increased its overall matriculation from 180 medical students to 210 students annually. The inaugural class of Temple/St. Luke's graduated in May 2015. In October 2015, TUSM changed its name to the Lewis Katz School of Medicine at Temple University (LKSOM).

St. Luke's has an unwavering commitment to excellence in patient care: to educate physicians, nurses, and other health care providers; and to improve access to care in the communities we serve. Temple/St. Luke's is a central part of our mission to train the next generation of physicians who will serve the Lehigh Valley and communities across the country. It is also a key to St. Luke's vision of increasing access, and ease of access, to health care.

Structure, Governance and Funding:

Temple/St. Luke's students spend their first year at LKSOM's Philadelphia campus. They then move to the Temple/St. Luke's campus in

Bethlehem for years two, three, and four. Temple/St. Luke's accepts 30 students per year, which corresponds to the number of students in one Doctoring College at LKSOM. The Doctoring Colleges are small learning groups within LKSOM that span all four years of school. All Temple/St. Luke's students belong to the Saunders Doctoring College, named for Charles D. Saunders, M.D., a skillful and compassionate physician who has practiced at St. Luke's for more than four decades and served in several leadership positions. The campus has its own Senior Associate Dean, Assistant Dean for Student Affairs, Director of Student Affairs, Director of Development, and Director of Simulation. The students are represented by elected Student Government Association (SGA) Representatives.

Student Body:

To be considered for Temple/St. Luke's, candidates must first apply to LKSOM through the American Medical College Application Service (AMCAS®). Candidates are then emailed with instructions for accessing the online supplemental application. When completing the supplemental application, interested candidates select Temple/St. Luke's as their first choice in the clinical/regional campus section. If invited to interview for the Temple/St. Luke's program, a candidate will participate in all the interview day activities at St. Luke's. We also encourage applicants to the Temple/St. Luke's program to tour LKSOM's Philadelphia campus. Admissions decisions are made on a rolling basis and interviewed applicants generally receive the admission committee's decision four to six weeks after the interview. Accepted students may be invited to attend Second Look Days at both the Bethlehem and Philadelphia campuses. At Temple/St. Luke's, Second Look Day provides applicants the chance to further explore our campus and the Lehigh Valley, meet some of their prospective classmates, and get answers to their questions, both during organized sessions and through informal conversations.

Agreements between LKSOM, St. Luke's, Lehigh University, Moravian College, Muhlenberg College, and De Sales University allow outstanding undergraduates from these schools to be considered at the end of their junior year as part of an Early Assurance Program (EAP). By the end of their junior year, EAP candidates must have completed the minimum science prerequisites and achieved at least a 3.6 GPA (overall and science), as well as having demonstrated a strong commitment to service with extensive community and healthcare experiences. Once accepted to the program, students take the MCAT exam by the end of May of their junior year. Subsequently, they must complete their senior year. Besides the EAP and the regular admissions program, Temple/St. Luke's also has an Early Decision Program open to both Pennsylvania and non-Pennsylvania residents.

Curriculum:

LKSOM has an integrated curriculum divided into interdisciplinary blocks organized according to organ systems. During their first year, students study the normal structure and function of each organ system. In their second year, students focus on disease processes of each organ system as well as learning therapeutic options to treat the diseases of the organ system.

In their second year, the integrated curriculum in Bethlehem is taught by St. Luke's pathologists, microbiologists, pharmacists, and various specialty clinicians. The subject matter is the same at both campuses and the students are evaluated using the same exams and other metrics.

During the first two years, students learn the culture and practice of medicine through Saunders Doctoring College. They learn the basics of history taking and clinical skills and participate in programs on professionalism, communication skills, ethics, and medical economics, as well as diversity and cultural competencies. Students learn on simulators, with standardized patient encounters, as well as from real patients.

In their third and fourth years, Temple/St. Luke's students rotate through various required clinical services and have over five months of elective time. Electives can be taken anywhere within the Temple University Health System. Students may take two outside electives, as well as one international elective.

Throughout the curriculum, students are exposed to several threads, including: population health, social determinants of health, patient-centered care, communication challenges, evidence-based medicine, patient safety, quality improvement, professionalism, and ethics. Students also work with other healthcare professionals, including nurses, physician assistants, and various technologists, which prepares them for the team-based, interprofessional environment of modern healthcare.

Unique Characteristics:

Temple/St. Luke's has an intimate, interactive learning environment. Workshops and other small group activities typically involve six or fewer students, and most clinical rotations involve no more than six to eight students at a time, ensuring that everyone can participate fully. The high ratio of attending physicians and residents to students affords unparalleled opportunities to learn.

Since all required third- and fourth-year rotations are at the same hospital, students are not required to master multiple computer systems and hospital layouts. Spending three years at Temple/St. Luke's provides students with the unique opportunity to build long-term relationships with attending physicians and residents, to assist with longitudinal research studies, and to become involved in the community.

Accomplishments and Challenges:

Students at the regional campus have performed comparably to the students at the main campus on examinations. At both campuses, first-time pass rates for USMLE Step One and Two are equal. Temple/St. Luke's graduates have been very successful in obtaining residency positions, and have also conducted research projects resulting in publications and presentations.

Future Plans:

The faculty are working together to decrease the number of hours students at both campuses spend in traditional lectures and increase time spent engaged in more interactive learning, including workshops and clinical reasoning conferences. We also have a goal of increasing interprofessional education. At Temple/St. Luke's, we plan to increase future class sizes and continue to build our relationships with the community.

10. Texas Tech University Health Sciences Center School of Medicine, Permian Basin

Authors:

- C. Neal Ellis, M.D.,
  Professor and Regional Chairman of Surgery,
  Program Director, Surgical Residency Program, Permian Basin,
  Texas Tech University Health Sciences Center
  School of Medicine, Permian Basin

- Valerie Bauer, M.D.,
  Associate Professor and Chief of Division of
  Colorectal Surgery, Surgery Clerkship Director,
  Third and Fourth Year Medical Students,
  Texas Tech University Health Sciences Center
  School of Medicine, Permian Basin

Regional Campus:

Texas Tech University Health Sciences Center
School of Medicine, Permian Basin
Location: Odessa, Texas

Institution (main campus):

Texas Tech University Health Sciences Center
School of Medicine, Lubbock
Location: Lubbock, Texas

History and Mission:

The Texas Tech University School of Medicine was established by the 61st State Legislature in 1969, creating a multi-campus institution to address a physician shortage in West Texas. The administrative center was built in Lubbock, adjacent to the Texas Tech University campus. Regional Medical Campuses followed in Amarillo, El Paso, and Permian Basin in strategically positioned locations across a vast terrain, spanning a 131,000 square mile area with over 2.7 million people.

The school expanded in 1979 to form the Texas Tech University Health Sciences Center (TTUHSC), with a charter to provide educational training for healthcare professionals in multiple disciplines. This includes academic programs in Allied Health and Biomedical Sciences, Medicine, Nursing, and Pharmacy. In 2013, TTUHSC-El Paso separated from TTUHSC, leaving Amarillo and Permian Basin as regional centers.

The goals of the regional campus were to:

- Address physician shortages and health disparities in rural West Texas by training graduates who stay to practice in the area;

- Provide quality educational opportunities in multiple academic programs;

- Advance knowledge through innovative scholarship and research, and provide exceptional patient care and services within the geographic region;

- Establish partnerships with clinical affiliates to enhance delivery of healthcare, research, and specialty care in rural West Texas.

Odessa was chosen to be the southernmost regional campus in 1978. Located 100 miles from Lubbock, and a two-hour drive through a rural landscape of cotton fields and oil wells, the city won its petition for the Regional Academic Health Center (RAHC) after demonstrating a strong community commitment to the institution. From its creation by the Legislature in 1969 to its official launch in 1986, it took 17 years to open. A chronology of highlights in its development and growth are summarized below:

1974- Affiliation agreement signed with Ector County hospital. Approval of $20.4 million dollars to upgrade hospital.

1978- Odessa named as site for RAHC based on citizen support: Chamber of Commerce petition of 22,000 signatures; $325,000 pledge for development; 292 hours per week pledged in volunteered teaching time by physicians.

1981- Ector County donated 6.1 acres for RAHC. Odessa surgeon, named as first (interim) associate dean.

1983- Texas Tech University regents approved $2.5 million for the RAHC. First official associate dean named.

1984- Groundbreaking ceremonies held. Accreditation of **Family Medicine Residency Program.**

1986- Regional campus opened.

1988- Accreditation of **OB/GYN Residency Program.**

1992- Accreditation of **Internal Medicine Residency Program.**

2009- Third year medical students began clinical training at regional campus.

2015- Accreditation of **Surgical Residency Program**.

2016- Accreditation of **Psychiatry Residency Program**.

2016- Rural hospitals partnered with regional campus to support training of surgical residents in rural medicine with support of state educational grants.

2018- Multiple specialty fellowships added, including programs in **Emergency Medicine, Endocrinology, Geriatric Medicine, Hospitalists Medicine, and Child and Adolescent Psychiatry**.

Structure, Governance and Funding:

Administrative governance and authority of the medical school is in Lubbock and under the full responsibility of the Dean, as Chief Academic Officer, for all academic and clinical programs offered by the campuses at Amarillo and Odessa. The Dean is directly responsible to the President of Texas Tech University Health Sciences Center, who, in turn, reports to the Chancellor, the Chief Executive Officer of the health system. The Chancellor and the President are responsible to the Board of Regents. The Regional Deans of Medicine are responsible to the Dean of the School of Medicine in Lubbock.

Funding comes primarily from revenue generated by professional services, state appropriations, and contracts/grants received from federal, state, local, and private sectors. Funding unique to the regional campus comes from affiliates who support resident and faculty salaries, including Ector County hospital and several other private and rural hospitals in the region.

Student Body:

The regional campus in Permian Basin began accepting third-year medical students in 2009, and has grown to currently include 25 students per class of third- and fourth-year students. This represents 14 percent of the class distribution, which was recently increased from 150 to 180 per class by the Liaison Committee on Medical Education. Applicants from West Texas and rural communities are strongly recruited, because they are more likely to return home to practice after graduation.

Third- and fourth-year students come to the regional campus after completing two years of basic science in Lubbock. They have four campuses from which they may choose to complete their clinical rotations: Lubbock (University Medical Center or Covenant Healthcare Systems), Amarillo, or the Permian Basin. Of these, Permian basin is the smallest, offering smaller class sizes, but more direct contact with teaching faculty and residents, and a community focus that may foster interest in primary care and/or practice in underserved areas.

Approximately half of medical school graduates remain in Texas to complete residency training, and nearly 20 percent stay in a TTUHSC residency program. Just over 50 percent of graduates elect primary care specialties, with nearly 30 percent of these staying in Texas, and over five percent practicing in underserved areas within the state.

Curriculum:

The clerkship experience is uniform across all campuses based on institutionally defined goals and objectives. The Clinical Education Operations Committee (CEOC) monitors content within and across the third- and fourth-year clerkships, and participates in a monthly curriculum review process that oversees measures of cross-campus comparability. This is attended by Clerkship Directors from all campuses via a teleconferencing link.

All clerkships utilize a standard series of assessment methodologies for determining student grades, including an NBME® subject exam, a common student performance assessment by faculty and residents, use of identical standardized patient encounters, and a shared set of required clinical experiences.

A longitudinal integrated program exists within the traditional block rotation, allowing students to follow patients in different clinical settings as opportunities arise. Dual degree programs in Medicine and Business Administration or Law are also available at the regional campus.

The Family Medicine Accelerated Track (FMAT) Program, an innovative fast-track medical education program that was the first of its kind, began in 2011. Developed to prepare primary care physicians more efficiently and with less cost, it combines a three-year medical degree with a three-year family medicine residency, allowing students to complete training in six years rather than seven.

Unique Characteristics:

The Family Medicine Rural Track is a distinctive program in primary care offered at the Permian Basin campus. Residents selected for this track work individually with a family physician practicing full-spectrum care, including: general and preventative medicine, operative procedures, surgical obstetrics and Texas-Mexico "border medicine". These residents spend two years in rural practices outside of Odessa.

The TTUHSC Laura W. Bush Institute for Women's Health was founded in 2007 to promote research, education, and community support programs specific to women's health. One of the regional centers is in Midland, where students and residents rotate to learn about delivery of gender-related healthcare in this community.

Students and residents interested in research or outreach projects related to rural health are supported through The F. Marie Hall Institute for Rural and Community Health. The institute supports the advancement of health through imaginative and scholarly research, innovative use of technology, comprehensive education, and outreach.

Accomplishments and Challenges:

More than 20 percent of the practicing physicians in West Texas graduated from the TTUHSC School of Medicine and/or residency programs, many of whom received part or all of their training at the regional campus in Permian Basin. The earlier physician to resident ratio of 1:1,300 has decreased by nearly half, down to 1:700 with the development of the medical school throughout West Texas. In addition, the AAMC Graduate Questionnaire indicates that our students have consistently "agreed or strongly agreed" that they are satisfied with their medical education at Permian Basin.

Recruiting faculty physicians represents one of the greatest challenges for our campus due to the high cost of housing in an area where real estate is inflated by the oil industry. Similarly, competitive applicants for administrative and staff positions are also lured away by higher paying positions in the oil industry. Maintaining adequate staffing of both faculty and administrative support is of paramount importance in a rapidly growing regional medical campus.

Future Plans:

The regional campus in Odessa will continue to expand both undergraduate and graduate medical education and training programs for medical students and residents. Long term plans include further development of basic science and clinical research programs, as well as further diversification of academic opportunities.

References:

1. The Odessa American (Odessa, Texas) · Sat, Nov 6, 1982

2. *Texas Tech University Health Sciences Center Fact Book*, 24th edition. December, 2017 Prepared by the Office of the Vice President and Chief Financial Officer.

3. *STATE OF TEXAS LEGISLATIVE APPROPRIATIONS REQUEST For Fiscal Years 2018 and 2019*, Submitted to the Office of the Governor, Budget Division and the Legislative Budget Board, Texas Tech University Health Sciences Center October 17, 2016.

11. The University of Oklahoma-Tulsa (OU-TU) School of Community Medicine

Authors:

- Brent W. Beasley, M.D.,
  MBA, Professor of Medicine,
  The OU-TU School of Community Medicine

- Meredith Davison, Ph.D., MPH,
  Associate Dean of Academic Services,
  Associate Program Director, Physician's Assistant Program,
  The OU-TU School of Community Medicine

Regional Campus:

The University of Oklahoma-Tulsa (OU-TU)
School of Community Medicine
Location: Tulsa, Oklahoma

Institution (main campus):

The University of Oklahoma College of Medicine
Location: Oklahoma City, Oklahoma

History and Mission:

In 1972, the Oklahoma Legislature authorized The University of Oklahoma College of Medicine (OUCOM), located 103 miles away in Oklahoma City (OKC), to establish a Regional Medical Campus (RMC) in Tulsa to train more providers for Northeastern Oklahoma, and to provide healthcare for uninsured patients in the region[1]. The new funding allowed for 30 medical students in each class to spend their clinical rotations on the Tulsa campus.

Over the next 25 years, 60 third- and fourth-year medical students worked with full-time faculty and residents in each of six specialties: Internal Medicine, Family Medicine, Obstetrics and Gynecology, Pediatrics, General Surgery, and Psychiatry. A large and diverse group of volunteer specialty faculty precepted students in the hospitals, and in their private outpatient clinics. The campus built a strong community sense of responsibility to train the next generation of physicians.

In 1999, The Charles and Lynn Schusterman Family Foundation donated 60 acres in mid-Tulsa to upgrade the OU-Tulsa campus: new administrative and education buildings, a library, a simulation center, and a $30 million-dollar clinic. OU consolidated their Tulsa area healthcare education and training programs on the new Schusterman Center campus, decreasing education costs by sharing resources.

The OUCOM rebranded the Tulsa campus in 2008 as The University of Oklahoma *School of Community Medicine* (SCM). A $50 million gift from the George Kaiser Family Foundation established a mission to improve the health and healthcare of the entire community.[1] In 2015, the SCM welcomed its first complement of 26 first-year medical students, and with succeeding classes completed its expansion to include a total of 120 students in the four-year Tulsa curriculum.

Structure, Governance and Funding:

The OUCOM has a centralized governance structure covering the medical school on both campuses, in Oklahoma City and in Tulsa. The oversight of the curriculum is the responsibility of the Executive Dean and the Faculty Board. Three curriculum committees oversee development and evaluation:

- The Preclinical Science Education Committee is responsible for the first two years.

- The Clinical Science Education Committee is responsible for the last two years. The Clerkship Directors in Tulsa have equal voting with the OKC Clerkship Directors.

- A Medical Education Committee coordinates the first two committees to ensure integration and oversight of the educational program.

The Dean of OU-Tulsa reports to the OUCOM Executive Dean for the medical school curriculum and the OU Provost for other activities (i.e. physician group and GME). Funding for the OU-Tulsa campus comes from state appropriations, tuition, clinical revenue, hospitals, and grants from philanthropies.

Student Body:

Students wishing to attend OU-Tulsa apply to OUCOM and then to the SCM. They must be acceptable to the faculty on both campuses. Students chosen for the SCM must demonstrate interest in public health, community medicine, and underserved populations.

- The OU-Tulsa SCM student body hails primarily from Oklahoma (90 percent) with less than 5 percent of Native American heritage.

- Approximately 40 percent of the OU-Tulsa SCM students choose primary care specialties.

- Approximately 10 to 20 percent of the OU-Tulsa SCM remain in Tulsa for residency, and 10 to 20 percent go to OKC, although this fluctuates yearly.

- An internal study showed approximately 65 percent of OU-Tulsa SCM students practice in Oklahoma after training.

Curriculum:

The first two years of morning didactics are video-conferenced and recorded between the campuses, 75 percent originating from OKC, and 25 percent from Tulsa. The curriculum model is competency-based around organ systems, integrated to emphasize connections between basic and clinical sciences.

Team-based learning is used throughout the first two years.[2] For instance, the Clinical Medicine Course includes Standardized Patient Based Learning exercises quarterly. A team of learners interviews and examines standardized patients with common ambulatory complaints. The team creates a differential diagnosis and researches the potential diseases to determine the most likely diagnoses and treatment options. The exercise culminates with presentations in front of primary care physicians.

The third- and fourth-year medical student rotations are required to remain comparable between the two campuses, understanding that the two experiences will not be identical. The curricula for each clinical rotation are organized around six general competencies: Practice-Based Learning and Improvement, Patient Care and Procedural Skills, Systems-Based Practice, Medical Knowledge, Interpersonal and Communication Skills, and Professionalism. In addition, the SCM students learn a "7th Competency of Community Medicine," including objectives related to population medicine, public health, and social determinants of health.

Innovative Curricular Offerings:

1. Summer Institute is a four-day interdisciplinary immersion curriculum in community medicine for new health professions students. They take part in a variety of innovative experiences, including group interviews with patients and a family-in-poverty simulation. They also learn about healthcare delivery and inequities, the "anatomy" of the Tulsa community, and social determinants of health.[3]

2. Since 2003, the Bedlam Clinic, a student-run free clinic set up for health professions students, provides hands-on experience to gain practical healthcare skills. Medical students participate in this clinic during all four years.

3. Third-year students also participate in Bedlam Longitudinal clinic, providing primary care to their own continuity panel of approximately 15 to 20 chronically ill uninsured patients under faculty supervision two afternoons per month.

4. "Student Academy" occurs one Friday per month for OU-Tulsa third-year medical students and second-year physician assistant students, covering educational topics related to the most common

problems seen in the Bedlam Clinic. In the morning, faculty provide case presentations based on the students' readings, and students use Problem-based Learning to arrive at diagnoses and treatments. Procedural skill sessions and small group ethics discussions occur in the afternoons in the $6.4 million, 16,000-square-foot Tandy Education Center simulation laboratory.

5. Students have the opportunity to be involved in a variety of health advocacy experiences. This last year, a group of students worked with the Tulsa County Medical Society to encourage state legislators to pass a new law preventing minors from participating in tanning salons.

6. An Ultrasound course began with second-year students in Tulsa as "voluntary sessions" during evenings. After great turnout and success, a formalized Ultrasound curriculum was added at both campuses — a good example of how Tulsa has been a curriculum laboratory for the entire medical school.

Unique Characteristics:

7. Approximately 20 percent of Tulsa students enroll in the combined MD/MPH program, a five-year track that includes an extra year between the second and third year of medical school. Tuition for the MPH degree is covered by scholarship funds.

8. All of the SCM medical students participate in the Bedlam Clinic (see above) to work with other providers and faculty to provide walk-in services to patients without insurance.

Accomplishments and Challenges:

The OU Tulsa SCM produces a large number of MD/MPH students, who have an enhanced understanding of population medicine as they begin practice. Additionally, current data suggests SCM students are more knowledgeable about public health issues and disparities than other medical students, and have more positive attitudes toward underserved populations. We anticipate this will translate into physicians better able to serve diverse patient populations. Our challenges are most often related to adequate funding for unique programs.

Future Plans:

- OU Health System plans clinical integration between OKC and Tulsa campuses, including a common EMR, co-branding, co-marketing, and co-contracting.

- OU Tulsa SCM anticipates a change from a weak partnership with several Tulsa hospitals to an interconnected relationship with one or two hospitals dedicated to an academic mission.

- We plan to increase access to our faculty physicians by expanding our health system locations throughout the region, reaching all segments of the community, and broadening our focus beyond the underserved.

- We also expect to expand the medical school class size as we move forward.

12. Tufts University School of Medicine Maine Medical Center Program

Authors:

- Jo Ellen Linder, M.D.,
  Associate Professor, Department of Emergency Medicine
  and Department of Public Health & Professional
  Degree Programs, Director of Student Affairs,
  Tufts University School of Medicine Maine Medical Center Program

- Sarah Couser MS IV,
  Tufts University School of Medicine Maine Medical Center Program

Regional Campus:

> Tufts University School of Medicine
> Maine Medical Center Program
> **Location:** Portland, Maine

Institution (main campus):

> Tufts University School of Medicine
> **Location:** Boston, Massachusetts

History and Mission:

Tufts University School of Medicine was founded in April 1893, the initial graduate degree program at Tufts College. Maine Medical Center has a long-established commitment to medical education, training an increasing number of residents and fellows since the middle of the last century. In 2006, a medical education strategic planning process resulted in several strategic goals, including: to *improve access to medical school for qualified Maine residents and to help address the workforce needs throughout the state in all specialties.* Tufts University School of Medicine Maine Medical Center Program (TUSM-MMC) aka the "Maine Track" established a new innovative model to teach medical students starting in 2009. Tufts Health Sciences campus is 110 miles from Maine Medical Center with travel between the two primary campus sites taking two hours by auto, bus, or train. The mission: Maine Medical Center and Tufts University School of Medicine jointly commit to developing and implementing a unique medical school program, featuring an innovative curriculum that will offer both tertiary-care and rural-based experiences in Maine, train exceptional physicians, and encourage graduates to pursue career opportunities in Maine.

Structure, Governance and Funding:

The Maine Track program is anchored in the Department of Medical Education at Maine Medical Center, located in Portland, Maine. The Academic Dean in Maine is the Senior Vice President for Academic Affairs. The Maine Track Steering Committee is co-chaired by TUSM Dean and MMC President & CEO and includes leaders from both the Boston and Maine campuses. Additional Maine committees and subcommittees include faculty and staff who serve as course directors, clerkship site directors, preceptors, formal advisors, and informal mentors. Rural teaching sites include TUSM-MMC Rural Longitudinal Integrated Clerkship sites and community practices that provide clinical experiences for students in primary care and several specialties. Several sources of funding support the programs, including a multi-million dollar philanthropic effort that supports student scholarships each year. Modest support from grants and from Tufts provide some funding for the program, however rural LIC sites bear most of the program costs including student housing.

Student Body:

Up to 40 students are admitted to the Maine Track each year, comprising approximately 20 percent of the Tufts class of 200. The majority of Maine Track students are from Maine or have some ties to Maine through family or education. All candidates submit their applications through the TUSM Admissions online application process. Members of the Maine Track Admissions subcommittee interview qualified applicants in Portland blending standard interviews and multiple mini-interview stations. Maine Track mission-based admissions decisions are made on a rolling basis in Maine with final decisions made by Tufts Admissions Committee. Student body diversity is enhanced with students from rural communities and those who are underrepresented in medicine. Approximately half of the Maine Track graduates match in primary care specialties (family medicine, internal medicine, pediatrics). As of fall 2017, 13 Maine Track alumni are practicing family medicine, internal medicine, emergency medicine, and obstetrics and gynecology in six different counties.

Curriculum:

TUSM-MMC started in 2009 when a revised curriculum was being implemented at Tufts. The Maine Track curriculum builds on Tufts competency-based curriculum and incorporates Maine's unique concepts and problems. Students are placed based on their preferences at several teaching sites ranging from integrated health systems to small community primary care practices, Federally Qualified Health Centers, critical access hospitals, and Veterans Administration clinical sites.

Although most of first and second year are spent in Boston, Maine track students matriculate in Maine and spend approximately 10 days in an experiential orientation that includes workshops, team-building on an island, and team-based care activities in both a Maine community and tertiary care center. All Tufts students are assigned to a primary care preceptor for the *Competency-based Apprenticeship in Primary Care (CAP)* starting at the end of first year and extending through second year. CAP preceptors for Maine Track Students are located in Maine.

Figure 1. Most of the Maine Track students complete their core clerkships in the Longitudinal Integrated Curriculum (LIC) Model at one of eleven LIC sites. Maine Track students must complete at least five fourth- year advanced rotations in Maine. Several four-week clinical electives are offered at rural and smaller community teaching sites around the state. Maine Track students may also participate in Global Health experiences during the summer between first and second year and spring semester of fourth year, funded primarily by TUSM Office of Minority Affairs and Global Health. Up to five TUSM-MMC students complete the MD-MPH dual degree program within four years.

Unique Characteristics:

The Maine Track features meaningful exposure to clinical practice in rural communities, with opportunities offered throughout all four years. Rural LIC experiences over nine months has energized and engaged entire healthcare systems in small communities throughout the state. The LIC Director in Norway, Maine stated, "Our critical access hospital has truly become an academic medical center where everyone feels committed to teaching Tufts Maine Track students." The Certificate in Health Care Improvement course, initiated in AY17-18, combines local teams at some LIC sites working with experts onsite, as well as through distance learning. MMC Department of Medical Education offers a fourth-year enrichment elective in Medical Education. A Wilderness Medicine elective, taught by Emergency Medicine TUSM-MMC faculty, is offered in the last block of fourth year. Capstone is a one-week course, led by MMC's Director of Fourth Year, and offered at the end of fourth year as a preparation for residency, incorporating clinical skills workshops and hi-fidelity simulation cases.

Accomplishments and Challenges:

Ongoing assessments of the innovative Maine Track curriculum have resulted in several publications. A number of Maine physicians have been recognized each year with faculty awards in Maine and at Tufts. Two student-led programs include service to underserved, vulnerable populations in rural *(Sipayik Reservation)* and urban settings *(Preble Street Learning Collaborative)*. The Rural Internal Medicine in Maine *(RIMM)* graduate medical education program at Stephens Memorial Hospital grew out of a desire to add graduate medical education (GME) at the rural LIC site. *RIMM* welcomed the first internal medicine resident in July 2017.

A primary challenge of the curriculum is the several moves Maine Track students make during medical school. Housing has been provided to students during first and second year when students are in Maine for orientation and required courses. Cost of student housing at rural LIC sites has been borne by the hospitals and is becoming more burdensome. Efforts to reduce student debt through scholarships and covering some expenses helped to reduce overall student debt, however the high cost of tuition and expenses remain challenging.

Future Plans:

TUSM faculty adopted a new educational strategic plan and began work to implement a comprehensive curriculum revision starting with the incoming class in AY 2019-2020. At the same time, TUSM-MMC plans to expand pre-clinical required courses offered in Maine in the end of first year and all of second year. Graduate Medical Education expansion to additional rural sites beyond the *RIMM* program is a long-range plan.

13. UCSF Fresno Medical Education Program

Authors:

- Kenny Banh, M.D.,
  Assistant Dean of Undergraduate Medical Education (UME);
  Associate Professor of Clinical Emergency Medicine;
  UCSF Fresno Medical Education Program

- Loren I. Alving, M.D., HS
  Clinical Professor of Neurology,
  Curriculum Director SJV PRIME,
  UCSF Fresno Medical Education Program

Regional Campus:

UCSF Fresno Medical Education Program
Location: Fresno, California

Institution (main campus):

University of California, San Francisco (UCSF)
School of Medicine
Location: San Francisco, California

History and Mission:

University of California San Francisco was established in 1864 as Toland Medical College, became affiliated with the University of California in 1873, and was designated as the UC Medical Center in San Francisco in 1949.

Fresno, 180 miles southeast of San Francisco, and the surrounding central San Joaquin Valley is one of the poorest areas in the country. In 1970, it was identified by the Carnegie Commission as being underserved in medicine, which led to the creation of the San Joaquin Valley Health Consortium to address disparities in health care, notably the physician shortage. Efforts by this group and the University of California led to the establishment of an Area Health Education Center (AHEC) in Fresno in 1972, followed in 1975 by the establishment of the UCSF Fresno Medical Education Program (MEP), with support from a California Assembly Resolution, as well as funds and participation from Fresno Veterans Administration Medical Center (VAMC) and Valley Medical Center (VMC). The stated goal was to address the regional shortage by training family physicians and other primary care physicians.

Initially, the UCSF Fresno MEP was housed at the Fresno VAMC, transitioning to the current location at the Community Regional Medical Center campus in 2005.

In 2009, the Central Valley Program in Medical Education was established as a collaboration between UC Davis School of Medicine, UCSF, UC Merced, and UCSF Fresno, with funding from the California Legislature, resulting in the San Joaquin Valley Programs in Medical Education program (SJV PRIME) to train more doctors who want to work in the San Joaquin Valley.

Structure, Governance, and Funding:

We have an Associate Dean of the UCSF Fresno MEP who reports directly to the Vice Dean of Medical Education at the main campus. Recently we added an Assistant Dean of Undergraduate Medical Education as our program has expanded.

We have three major sources of funding. Initially, our funds came out of the general regional campus MEP budget. In 2009 SJV PRIME was established, which provided additional funding for students from California. More recently we began receiving Professional Degree Supplemental Tuition (PDST) funds.

Student Body:

We have two sets of students: those doing traditional rotations (core third-year clerkships and fourth-year rotations) and SJV PRIME students.

Medical students have been rotating on a case-by-case basis since the early 1970s. By 1980, core third-year clerkship opportunities existed for UCSF students in Family Medicine, OB/GYN, and Psychiatry; clerkships in Neurology, Surgery, and Pediatrics followed. Currently, students from UCSF and UC Davis can rotate in all core clerkships; students from these and other campuses participate in fourth-year elective clerkships.

UC PRIME programs exist at several UC campuses to meet the needs of California's underserved urban and rural populations. SJV PRIME, established in 2009, is not specifically a rural, primary care, or Latino program. Students are selected from those admitted to the UC Davis School of Medicine based on the strength of their ties to the Central

Valley and commitment to underserved medicine and improving health disparities. Students from the class of 2013 joined our campus in 2011, and since then, compared with students who rotated through Fresno in the past, the SJV PRIME students have been drawn from much more demographically diverse backgrounds: 70 percent are first-generation college students and identify as socioeconomically disadvantaged, and approximately half are from underrepresented minorities.

SJV PRIME students do their two preclinical years at UC Davis, their third year at UCSF Fresno, and their fourth year at any combination of the two. They participate in a pre-matriculation program at UC Merced in July of their entering year and have the opportunity to participate in the REACH (Research, Education and Community Health) program in Fresno and Merced (see below) between their first and second years.

By June 2018, SJV PRIME will have graduated 25 students, with 68 percent entering residencies in potential primary care tracks.

Curriculum:

Traditional block rotations for UCSF and UC Davis students are coordinated by local clerkship directors. Ultimate oversight rests with the academic faculty at each institution.

SJV PRIME students are enrolled in traditional block rotations for OB/GYN and Surgery. They participate in an expanded version of the outpatient-based Longitudinal Integrated Curriculum (LIC), originally developed by UCSF Fresno for third-year UCSF students, which covers internal medicine, family medicine, psychiatry, neurology, and pediatrics. Doctoring (a physician skill development course) and an every-other-week educational half-day for the LIC are part of the required curriculum. The Fresno SJV PRIME clerkship director and individual local clerkship directors for each discipline coordinate the students' experience. Ultimate oversight, including grading and generation of MSPEs, is provided by clerkship directors and academic faculty at UC Davis in conjunction with the Fresno SJV PRIME clerkship director.

Unique Characteristics:

Research Education and Community Health (REACH) is a program offered between the first and second year developed by a group of then first-year students in 2015 who wanted more exposure and integration in the Fresno community prior to starting their third year. This program is a four-week class that includes clinical exposure in outpatient primary care, a research project, mentoring pre-med and disadvantaged high school students in the community, and first-hand education about underserved populations in the Valley.

Accomplishments and Challenges:

One of our biggest challenges has been to provide a core clerkship site for two different institutions. This entails not only different clerkship requirements, but different evaluation scales and forms, different demands for absences from clinical duties (because of longitudinal clerkships or doctoring sessions), and different calendars (different start dates, break times, and intersession dates).

We have had to provide more training for our attendings because of the confusion generated by the different evaluation scales. We have also had to work out the differences in the two schools' use of formative and summative grading, and we have tried to mirror their practical application of the grading scales so as not to under- or over-value our students. Site clerkship directors have worked with the clerkship directors at the respective schools to achieve parity.

UCSF's adoption of a new curriculum (Bridges) with one-day-a-week didactics during clinical rotations made differences in clerkship attendance quite evident. Ultimately, we have chosen to design our clerkships as much as possible so that student absences from clinical rotations to participate in other components of the curriculum will appear identical across campuses; the SJV PRIME students have a family medicine clinic and an education day on alternating weeks, which mirror the UCSF student absences.

In the coming year, the adoption of a new third-year calendar by UCSF will result in third-year students from UCSF and UC Davis with different amounts of clinical experience being together; this may be confusing for their attendings and will require faculty education.

Another challenge we face is consistently filling the SJV PRIME class, since students do not apply directly for admission to this track, but instead apply to the School of Medicine and then, if accepted, are considered for the program.

Future Plans:

Short-term plans include consolidating our program with UCSF: the SJV PRIME students entering Class of 2020, will be enrolled through UCSF.

Possible long-term plans include increasing the class size, ultimately to 50 students per year, and becoming a four-year Regional Medical Campus (RMC) of UCSF delivering both a preclinical and clinical curriculum.

14. University of Alabama at Birmingham, Huntsville Regional Medical Campus

Authors:

- Lanita S. Carter, Ph.D.,
  Director of Medical Education and Student Services,
  Assistant Professor, Department of Medical Education,
  University of Alabama at Birmingham,
  Huntsville Regional Medical Campus

- Paula Cothren, B.A.,
  Director of Academic Programs & Administrative Services,
  University of Alabama at Birmingham,
  Huntsville Regional Medical Campus

- Roger D. Smalligan, M.D., MPH,
  Regional Dean and Executive Director,
  Professor of Medicine,
  University of Alabama at Birmingham,
  Huntsville Regional Medical Campus

Regional Campus:

University of Alabama at Birmingham,
Huntsville Regional Medical Campus,
Location: Huntsville, Alabama

Institution (main campus):

> University of Alabama at Birmingham School of Medicine
> **Location:** Birmingham, Alabama

History and Mission:

The University of Alabama at Birmingham's (UAB) Huntsville Regional Medical Campus (HRMC) was established in 1971 as part of a medical education expansion for the State of Alabama. One goal of the expansion was to train and ultimately retain more physicians in underserved areas. To achieve this goal, the HRMC established a clinical campus for UAB third- and fourth-year medical students performing clerkships and electives emphasizing primary care. In addition, the Family Medicine residency program at Huntsville Hospital (36 residents) was established. It was the first approved and fully accredited Family Medicine residency in Alabama and is recognized as one of the premier Family Medicine residencies in the Southeast.

With campus growth, the Regional Dean recruited full-time teaching faculty in Family Medicine, Internal Medicine, Pediatrics, OB/GYN and Psychiatry, and formed a faculty practice plan. Part-time and volunteer community faculty were sought for other clerkships and, in 2012, a UAB Internal Medicine residency program (24 residents) was added. Furthermore, one-year fellowships in obstetrics and emergency medicine were developed at Huntsville Hospital.

Huntsville is located 100 miles north of the UAB campus and travel time between the two is less than two hours. Patient-care and teaching takes place in the UAB Medicine Huntsville clinics, community faculty private offices, at the 941-bed Huntsville Hospital (the primary teaching hospital), and other affiliated hospitals and clinics in the region.

Structure, Governance and Funding:

The Regional Dean oversees all clinical, educational, and research activities and reports regularly to the Dean of the UAB School of Medicine. The Regional Dean is supported locally by an Assistant Dean of Finance and Administration, a Director of Academic Programs and Administrative Services, a Director of Medical Education and Student Services, and a Finance Officer. On the academic side there are regional chairs of Family Medicine, Internal Medicine, Pediatrics, and Psychiatry, and part-time chairs of Neurology, OB/GYN, and Surgery. Funding includes state money from the main campus (26 percent), tuition (13 percent), and income generated by the faculty and residency practices in Huntsville, known as the Valley Foundation (59 percent), as well as local contracts (2 percent).

Student Body:

Upon entry to UAB, students can select where to do their clinical work. Anecdotal reports from previous HRMC students portray rich opportunities for working one-on-one with residents, attendings, and community physicians, making the Huntsville campus a popular choice for clinical rotations. Annually, there are 70 HRMC students (35 in each year) and they reflect the demographics of the school: 90 percent in-state and 10 percent out-of-state with 8 to 15 percent of students from under-represented minority groups. A recent change in admissions procedures now fills the HRMC class with a combination of voluntary and assigned students.

Although primary care is emphasized at the HRMC, students completing the program are qualified to enter residency in any discipline. Students with specific non-primary care specialty interests do away rotations during the fourth year.

Also upon entry, all students participate in Learning Communities comprised of 18 students and two faculty mentors based on their assigned campuses. This four-year longitudinal experience develops camaraderie among those joining together at the regional campus.

HRMC students perform well and typically match into one of their top three residency choices. Speciality choices over the past 10 years are illustrated below:

Huntsville Medical Student Internship Match Results 2006 to 2016

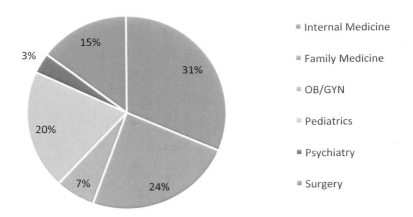

- Internal Medicine
- Family Medicine
- OB/GYN
- Pediatrics
- Psychiatry
- Surgery

Curriculum:

Third-year clinical education is organized into eight-week blocks and four-week sub-blocks. The fourth year consists of acting internships and elective courses in four-week and two-week intervals. HRMC students are directly supported by the Huntsville Office of Medical Student Services that oversees course scheduling, NBME shelf exam administration, and collection and reporting of grades. Students also receive academic and career counselling on the Huntsville campus.

In addition, the office coordinates a weekly Dean's Conference featuring speakers on clinical subjects, career choices, bioethics, and professional development. Dean's Conference allows students to interact and share ideas and suggestions outside their smaller clerkship groups and learning communities.

Unique Characteristics:

Office of Family Health Education and Research:

The Office for Family Health Education and Research (OFHER) conducts research that deals with the health care education of primary care physicians, as well as broader issues of state health policy, health access, and health manpower. The office oversees a "pipeline" concept for recruiting rural students into the medical profession; the Huntsville Rural Premedical Internship; and the Rural Medicine Program. Funding is from the Alabama Family Practice Rural Health Board through the Alabama Department of Public Health.

Huntsville Rural Premedical Internship Program (HRPI):

Each year, 15-16 college students from rural communities participate in a two-month program that introduces them to a career in medicine through shadowing, seminars on patient care, and field trips to rural community hospitals and rural industry to understand their health care needs. A total of 302 college interns have participated in HRPI since the program started in 1992. Of these, 272 have completed their undergraduate degrees.

- 65.1 percent have been accepted to medical school.
- 53.4 percent of graduates chose a primary care specialty.
- 60 percent of the practicing physicians are in Alabama.
- 33.7 percent practice in rural Alabama.

Huntsville Rural Medicine Program:

The Rural Medicine Program (RMP) is a five-year rural family medicine/primary care oriented curriculum within the regular medical school curriculum. Phase I is a pre-matriculation year at Auburn University. Phase II consists of the first two years of medical school on the Birmingham campus with additional RMP requirements. Phase III encompasses the third and fourth years of medical school (clinical sciences) at the HRMC along with additional curriculum requirements.

RMP applicants must meet the minimum requirements for regular admission and demonstrate specific characteristics, including a rural sense of place and self-motivation that predict their abilities to become outstanding rural physicians.

Since 2006 there have been 97 RMP students. Of those who have completed their training, all practice in Alabama with 53 percent in rural areas of Alabama.

Accomplishments and Challenges:

HRMC students' performance on USMLE Step 2 and their match results are on par with the main campus. Other accomplishments include the creation of: 1) the Dean's Conference; 2) co-enrolled, longitudinal courses for extra credit in topics such as bioethics, pharmacology, and medical Spanish; 3) expanded global health opportunities for students (Dominican Republic, Peru); 4) the encouragement of abstracts and poster presentations; and 5) the development of a Simulation Boot Camp for residents.

The campus has transitioned from total state support to one supported largely by the patient care revenue generated by the faculty. This has allowed a profit sharing arrangement with faculty and staff called Sharing In Success.

Future Plans:

In the short-term, the HRMC seeks to recruit additional full-time teaching faculty and community-faculty interested in teaching. It also strives to maintain excellent residency match outcomes for our graduating students and high board certification rates for our residents. Furthermore, the campus will encourage and reward scholarly activity, expand global health opportunities, and improve the social media presence for the campus and the clinics.

Long-term, the HRMC would like to expand overall class size, consider starting new residencies in our main hospital or at nearby rural hospitals, and increase the market share of primary care provided in our region.

15. University of Arkansas for Medical Sciences Northwest Arkansas Regional Campus (UAMS-NW)

Authors:

- Pearl Anna McElfish, Ph.D.,
  Associate Vice Chancellor, Assistant Professor,
  Department of Internal Medicine,
  University of Arkansas for Medical Sciences
  Northwest Arkansas Regional Campus

- Peter O. Kohler, M.D.,
  Distinguished Professor Emeritus, Department of
  Internal Medicine, Vice Chancellor (2007-2017),
  University of Arkansas for Medical Sciences
  Northwest Arkansas Regional Campus

- Thomas Schulz, M.D.,
  Interim Regional Associate Dean, Associate Professor,
  Department of Internal Medicine,
  Director of Internal Medicine Residency Program,
  University of Arkansas for Medical Sciences
  Northwest Arkansas Regional Campus

Regional Campus:

University of Arkansas for Medical Sciences
Northwest Arkansas Regional Campus (UAMS-NW)
Location: Fayetteville, Arkansas

Institution (main campus):

University of Arkansas for Medical Sciences (UAMS)
Location: Little Rock, Arkansas

History and Mission:

The University of Arkansas for Medical Sciences (UAMS) was founded in 1879 in the state capital of Little Rock, Arkansas, as the state's only medical school. In 1973, an Area Health Education Center (AHEC) was established in Fayetteville, Arkansas, offering primary care services and family medicine residency opportunities in the northwest region of the state. Because of concerns about a shortage of state health workers, and leveraging the presence of the AHEC, a regional campus of UAMS was established in northwest Arkansas in 2007. That same year, UAMS and Washington County agreed on a long-term lease for the regional campus. Academic units quickly followed with the College of Medicine in 2009, College of Pharmacy in 2011, and the College of Nursing in 2012. The College of Health Professions, which already had a radiology imaging sciences program in the AHEC, enhanced its presence with a doctorate of physical therapy program in 2014. Psychiatry and Internal Medicine residency programs have also been established. The Office of Community Health and Research, the campus research arm, began in 2014 and has earned more than $12 million in grants to date.

Funding and Governance:

In 2009, a tobacco tax was passed in Arkansas to fund several health-related projects. This has included building a statewide trauma network and supporting the UAMS Northwest Arkansas Regional Campus.

This tax-derived funding requires the campus to operate with a $3 million appropriation. The vice chancellor for UAMS Northwest Regional Campus reports to the UAMS chancellor, provides local leadership, and facilitates local strategy. Each of the academic programs has a regional associate dean or director. The regional associate dean of medicine is responsible for undergraduate and graduate medical education on the regional campus. The regional deans and directors of each academic program report to their respective deans and have a secondary reporting relationship for coordinated strategy, clinical, and research activities to the vice chancellor of the regional campus. A local executive committee of regional deans and directors works on joint projects such as interprofessional education. In addition, a local advisory board of community leaders facilitates local strategy and fundraising.

Student Body:

Currently, more than 250 students attend the regional medical campus (RMC) each year. The RMC educates approximately 36 third- and fourth-year medical students, approximately 60 third- and fourth-year pharmacy students, approximately 60 graduate nursing students, and approximately 105 health professions students. During the recruitment process, the opportunity to spend the third and fourth year on the regional campus is discussed. Once accepted for admission, students are required to choose a campus for third and fourth year. If too many or too few choose the regional campus, student allocation is chosen through a lottery process. Nursing and health profession students begin their education on the regional campus. UAMS is a three hour drive from the main campus in Little Rock, making virtual linkages very important. Many classes are shared between Little Rock and Fayetteville via interactive video connections. Classes are led from both the main UAMS campus in Little Rock and from UAMS Northwest Regional Campus. Graduation for all students is held on the main campus. Between 2009 and 2017, 336 doctors, nurses, pharmacists, and other health professionals have graduated from the UAMS Northwest Regional Campus.

Medical Curriculum:

The medical school utilizes a longitudinal integrated curriculum with third-year clerkship groups of surgery, internal medicine, neurology, pediatrics, obstetrics/gynecology, and psychiatry. The family medicine clerkship occurs through a weekly clinic experience throughout the entire year, allowing for continuity of patient care. In between the semesters is an "interphase" of four weeks in which students may complete elective experiences in radiology, otolaryngology, orthopaedics, and rehabilitation medicine. The fourth year is more traditional in layout, with block experiences in geriatrics, acting internships, medical and surgical subspecialty electives, and research. Clinical experiences are provided by community-based faculty at four local hospitals and other selected medical practices. Library and student services are provided through dedicated staff members who facilitate student activities across programs. The vast majority (more than 80 percent) of RMC graduates choose primary care (Family Medicine, Internal Medicine, Pediatrics, Med/Peds) for residency training.

Interprofessional Education and Research:

Because the UAMS Northwest Arkansas Regional Campus has students from multiple health professions, there is a unique opportunity to engage in inter-professional education and research. Educational activities include community health screenings, a student-led clinic, and seminars focused on reducing health disparities in diverse populations. Through the Office of Community Health and Research on the regional campus, the inter-professional activities have extended the opportunities for faculty, students, and residents across disciplines to conduct health disparities research and engage in scholarship. The campus uses a community-based participatory research (CBPR) approach. Research efforts have resulted in multiple extramural grants from the National Institutes of Health, Centers for the Disease Control and Prevention, and Patient Centered Outcomes Research Institute. The amount of scholarly activity increased by more than 300 percent since the Office of Community Health and Research was established, with more than 50 articles published by regional campus faculty and students between 2015 and 2017.

Accomplishments and Challenges:

Engaging community-based faculty to provide consistent preceptor sites continues to be the biggest challenge. To address this, the regional campus has recently established an Office of Community Based Faculty. In addition, campus leadership has identified the need for greater leadership development opportunities for faculty, residents, staff, and students. Leadership development programs are currently being planned. The campus has accomplished much in its first 10 years. Student test scores meet or exceed those at the main campus. All students have matched for residency. The CBPR program provides students, residents, and faculty a unique opportunity to engage in scholarship and has earned UAMS Northwest Regional Campus the 2017/2018 Star of Community Achievement Award given by the American Association of Medical Colleges' Group on Regional Medical Campuses.

Future Plans:

The northwest Arkansas community continues to call for an expanded presence of academic medicine in the region. In 2016, the local planning and business council, Northwest Arkansas Council, set a goal of making Northwest Arkansas a health care destination. As a result, the Northwest Arkansas Council has partnered with UAMS to determine the best growth plan for the regional campus. Possibilities include increasing the third- and fourth-year classes or potentially expanding the regional campus to a four-year medical school. In addition to the College of Medicine, the Colleges of Nursing, Pharmacy, and Health Professions are also planning to expand. There is additional discussion on how to grow graduate medical education programs at the regional campus (despite the residency cap on local hospitals). UAMS understands that the growth of academic and research programs must be built upon a robust clinical practice that provides an environment for medical education, and is exploring how best to accomplish this goal.

16. University of Colorado School of Medicine Colorado Springs Branch

Authors:

- Erik A. Wallace, M.D., FACP,
  Associate Dean for Colorado Springs Branch,
  Associate Professor of Medicine,
  University of Colorado School of Medicine
  Colorado Springs Branch

- Jason Hendrickson MS IV,
  University of Colorado School of Medicine
  Colorado Springs Branch

- Chad R. Stickrath, M.D., FACP,
  Assistant Dean for Education,
  Associate Professor of Medicine,
  University of Colorado School of Medicine
  Colorado Springs Branch

Regional Campus:

University of Colorado School of Medicine
Colorado Springs Branch
Location: Colorado Springs, Colorado

Institution (main campus):

University of Colorado School of Medicine,
Anschutz Medical Campus
Location: Aurora, Colorado

History and Mission:

The University of Colorado School of Medicine (CUSOM) was founded in 1883 and remains the only allopathic medical school in Colorado. Around 2010, CUSOM pursued expansion of its class size to address the growing physician shortage. Establishing a new Regional Medical Campus (RMC) was essential to provide these additional students with clinical training opportunities.

With a population of approximately 450,000, Colorado Springs is one of the largest cities in the United States without an academic medical center or medical school. In 2012, to support the expansion of medical education and address the local physician workforce shortage, 83 percent of voters approved a 40-year lease agreement between city-owned Memorial Hospital and University of Colorado Health (UCHealth) that created funding to establish a CUSOM branch campus in Colorado Springs.

In June 2013, CUSOM received approval from the LCME to expand its class size from 160 to 184 with the additional 24 students slated to complete their third-year core clinical experiences at the Colorado Springs Branch (CSB). The administration offices for the CSB, located on the University of Colorado at Colorado Springs (UCCS) campus, are approximately 60 miles from the main Anschutz Medical Campus in Aurora with an average commute time of 60-90 minutes.

In January 2014, the Associate Dean for Colorado Springs Branch was hired with a vision, "To develop 21st century physician leaders who will improve the health of the community." The first cohort of students was recruited in 2014 and began their core clinical experiences in April 2016. This first class matched into residencies and graduated in 2018.

Structure, Governance, and Funding:

The Associate Dean for the CSB reports directly to the Senior Associate Dean for Education at the Anschutz Medical Campus. Joining the Associate Dean at the branch are the Assistant Dean for Education, Director for Didactics and Longitudinal Curriculum, Director for Student Development, Director for Community Engagement, Associate Director for Education, Branch Coordinator, Student Coordinator, and nine Clinical Liaisons that represent all core clinical specialties during third year.

Funding to support the CSB and the expansion of the CUSOM class size on the main campus in years one and two comes from the lease agreement between Memorial Hospital and UC Health that provides $3 million of funding per year for 40 years. Although all CSB funding is provided by this lease agreement, CSB students work with faculty in UC Health facilities in addition to other private and military inpatient and outpatient locations throughout the community.

Student Body:

The CSB accepts up to 24 students per class to complete their third year core clinical experiences at the branch campus. Students indicate interest in the CSB after admission to CUSOM, and are invited by the Associate Dean to attend CSB Preview Day in April to visit the community and educational facilities, and to meet with students and faculty. Final selection of students by committee assessment of student interest, "fit", and chances for success at the CSB is completed prior to matriculation. Student specialty and career interests are not factors for selection. Approximately half of the students in each class have prior or current connections to the Colorado Springs community. Twenty-one students from the first cohort in the Class of 2018 successfully completed the core clinical year with ten applying for primary care specialties (internal medicine, family medicine, pediatrics, and obstetrics and gynecology).

Curriculum:

The Colorado Springs Mentored Integrated Clerkship (COSMIC) curriculum, a version of a Longitudinal Integrated Clerkship (LIC), for the core clinical year ensures that students achieve the same goals, objectives, and competencies, observe the same required clinical conditions, and are assessed in the same manner as all CUSOM students. Students complete experiences in ten clinical specialties, lead weekly didactics, take subject examinations, log patient encounters, and meet with faculty for academic and career advising. The year begins with eight one-week inpatient immersion experiences in six different specialties followed by LIC experiences in Emergency Medicine, Musculoskeletal Medicine, Neurology, Psychiatry, Family Medicine, Internal Medicine (inpatient and outpatient), Pediatrics, Obstetrics and Gynecology, and Surgery for the remaining 10 months. Students gain insight into patient-centered experiences by navigating healthcare systems and by following a panel of patients across specialties over multiple visits.

Clinical experiences are complemented by four hours of student-led didactics each week. Students lead up to four sessions per year and coordinate with faculty mentors to produce pre-session readings, quiz questions, and interactive, case-based didactic content. Physical exam, pathology, radiology, and high-value care components are threaded into didactic sessions.

Students receive performance feedback through formative assessments and quarterly clinical evaluations by faculty. NBME subject examinations or in-house examinations for each core clinical specialty are administered every two to four weeks, mostly in the second half of the year. Final grades for clinical experiences are assigned at the completion of the year by a grading committee which includes the clinical block director from the main campus, the corresponding CSB specialty liaison, CSB student coordinator, and CSB Assistant Dean for Education.

Fourth-year clinical electives are available at the CSB; however, students are not required to complete electives at the CSB and may choose to return to the main campus for fourth year.

Unique Characteristics:

In addition to COSMIC, students are required to design, complete, and present a quality improvement project in one of their clinical settings. Students also receive leadership training and are required to partner with community organizations to develop service-learning projects. Prior to second year, students can volunteer for the Poverty Immersion in Colorado Springs (PICOS), a two-day experiential program to learn how to empathize with and care for the local resource-limited population. A student-run free clinic provides healthcare to uninsured patients and clinical learning opportunities for CSB students across all four years. Students also have curricular and clinical experiences working with patients with intellectual and developmental disabilities.

Accomplishments and Challenges:

For the first two CSB student cohorts, donations provided each student with $5,000 per year annually to relieve them of $20,000 in educational debt. Efforts to raise additional scholarship funds from the community are ongoing and remain a challenge. As for performance, the first student cohort exceeded the national mean scores on all seven required NBME subject exams. Over 80 percent of faculty attended core faculty development sessions and about 90 percent of faculty were retained for the second cohort. Limited availability of faculty in some specialties (neurology, obstetrics and gynecology) due to physician shortages in the community make it challenging to place all students with individual educators, especially when faculty are no longer able to teach for personal or professional reasons.

Future Plans:

Given the saturation of learners in some clinical specialties, there are no immediate plans to expand the CSB class size beyond 24 students per year. However, CUSOM has initiated a curricular reform process that may present new opportunities for CSB students to become more engaged with their education, service, and research at the branch campus during times outside of the core clinical year. Given the growing physician workforce shortages in the community, healthcare systems may be interested in growing their educational partnerships with the CSB to encourage medical students to return and eventually practice in the local community.

17. University of Kansas School of Medicine-Salina

Authors:

- Erik Bowell, MS IV,
  University of Kansas School of Medicine-Salina

- William Cathcart-Rake, M.D.,
  Dean of Salina Campus; Clinical Professor of Medicine;
  University of Kansas School of Medicine-Salina

Regional Campus:

University of Kansas School of Medicine-Salina
Location: Salina, Kansas

Institution (main campus):

University of Kansas School of Medicine
Location: Kansas City, Kansas

History and Mission:

The University of Kansas, School of Medicine (KUSM) was officially established in 1905. KUSM initially provided instruction at Bell Memorial Hospital in Rosedale, a community located in Kansas City. In 1924, the school moved to its current location in Kansas City. KUSM has continuously granted the M.D. degree since it opened and is the only medical school in Kansas.

In 2009, KUSM addressed the significant shortage of physicians in rural areas of Kansas by proposing the creation of a new four-year Regional Medical Campus (RMC) in the north central Kansas community of Salina.

In 2010, the Liaison Committee for Medical Education (LCME) concluded that appropriate resources were available to proceed with establishing the Salina RMC.

Several factors contributed to LCME's favorable decision to establish the Salina RMC. First was the presence of a successful rural track program in Salina. The rural track allowed up to four students to complete their final 18 months of clinical training in a rural setting. Second was the presence of an established family medicine residency program in Salina (Smoky Hill Family Medicine Residency Program). Third was an extremely supportive and progressive Salina Regional Health Center (SRHC). Fourth was strong community support, adequate financial resources, adequate facilities, and supportive members of the local medical community.

KUSM-Salina accepted its inaugural class of eight students in July 2011, and has admitted eight students per year since 2011. With a total of 32 students, KUSM-Salina is the smallest four-year medical school campus in North America. Additionally, Salina is one of the smallest communities to host a four-year M.D. degree-granting medical school.

KUSM-Salina's primary mission is to increase the number of future physicians more likely to practice primary care medicine in rural and underserved areas of Kansas.

Structure, Governance, and Funding:

The chief administrative officer for KUSM-Salina is the campus Dean. The KUSM-Salina Dean answers to the Executive Dean on the main KUSM campus in Kansas City. Additional faculty and staff are comprised of:

1) A full-time Associate Dean of Foundational Sciences
2) A part-time Associate Dean of Clinical Experiences
3) A full-time Assistant Dean for Operations and Administration
4) A part-time Director of Medical Education
5) A part-time instructor in human anatomy and histopathology
6) Twenty-four local physicians representing various specialties, who are responsible for teaching and evaluating third- and fourth-year medical students. These core faculty members receive small stipends.
7) Three full-time support staff
8) Approximately 40 volunteer faculty members.

Faculty appointments and promotions are governed by the main campus. Salina faculty members participate in most KUSM faculty committees.

KUSM provides a significant portion (80 percent) of the budget for the Salina RMC, but additional funds are also provided by SRHC and various organizations within the local community in support of the mission to provide physicians for rural Kansas.

Student Body:

There is not a separate admission process for students wishing to attend KUSM-Salina. Students interested in attending KUSM-Salina submit their AMCAS application through the centralized admissions office on the main campus. A secondary application allows students to rank their campus preferences (Kansas City, Wichita, or Salina). The KUSM Admissions Committee makes the final decision as to what eight students are to be assigned to the Salina RMC.

Since inception, seven classes have matriculated at KUSM-Salina (a total of 56 students) — 28 males and 28 females. Four of the first 56 matriculants are from underrepresented minority populations. Ninety-one percent of matriculants are in-state students. Seventy-one percent of students are from rural communities, as defined by the U.S. Census Bureau.

While the Salina campus was created to help address the shortage of rural primary care physicians, students are encouraged to choose the career pathway best suited for them. Past graduates from KUSM-Salina have entered residency programs in various specialties including: family medicine, internal medicine, pediatrics, obstetrics and gynecology, orthopedic surgery, urology, and pathology.

Curriculum:

The curriculum at KUSM-Salina is identical to that on the main campus and the Wichita RMC. Foundational science lectures are delivered to Salina students by means of live, interactive television. The lectures are also digitally recorded and available as podcasts. In AY 2017-18 KUSM implemented a new curriculum that increased first- and second-year student engagement in the educational process through case-based small group activities. The first two years consist of nine integrated blocks organized around organ systems, each eight weeks in length. A week between each block is reserved for scholarly activity, enrichment activities, or remediation. The third year of the curriculum is comprised of six eight-week clinical clerkships which include Family and Community Health, Gender and Reproductive Health, Care of the Surgical Patient, Care of the Adult, Neural and Behavioral Health, and Infant, Child and Adolescent Health. In Year Four, a rural preceptorship, a critical care clerkship, and a sub-internship are the only required clerkships, leaving time for elective clerkships and the residency application process.

Unique Characteristics:

What makes KUSM-Salina truly unique is its size. Having only eight students per class provides an environment for a collaborative educational experience. During the majority of clinical clerkships, students work one-on-one with an attending physician, promoting significant hands-on rather than observational experiences. Additionally, students can easily and readily identify a physician mentor early in medical school and meet with this individual frequently. Finally, the small class size allows for a close-knit student body. It is possible to know and interact with each and every student and faculty/staff member on campus. Students typically spend a significant amount of time together in class, as well as outside class, participating in city recreational league sports and impromptu social gatherings that are inclusive of all students.

Accomplishments and Challenges:

KUSM-Salina is proud of the fact that all graduates have matched in their first choice of a residency specialty. KUSM-Salina is also proud that many KUSM-Salina students have engaged in scholarly activities, presenting papers and posters in regional, national, and international meetings, and co-authoring manuscripts accepted for publication in peer-reviewed journals. The success of Salina RMC prompted the KU School of Nursing to establish a regional nursing school campus in Salina in 2017.

Major challenges to our RMC include:

1) competition with the main campus for students;
2) recognition and promotion of local faculty for their educational endeavors; and
3) promoting scholarly activities for students and faculty.

Future Plans:

KUSM-Salina will be completing a new medical education building in the spring of 2018. This building will triple the available floor space and provide ample room for both the RMC and the new regional nursing campus. Consequently, increasing the number of medical students trained on the Salina RMC is a definite possibility.

18. University of Kentucky College of Medicine Rural Physician Leadership Program

Authors:

- Anthony Weaver, M.D.,
  Assistant Dean, Rural Physician Leadership Program,
  Associate Professor of Medicine,
  University of Kentucky, College of Medicine

- Megan Dillon MS IV,
  Rural Physician Leadership Program,
  University of Kentucky College of Medicine

Regional Campus:

University of Kentucky College of Medicine
Rural Physician Leadership Program
Location: Morehead, Kentucky

Institution (main campus):

University of Kentucky College of Medicine
Location: Lexington, Kentucky

History and Mission:

The University of Kentucky College of Medicine (UK COM) was established in 1960 in Lexington. Total enrollment is currently 547 students, with new four-year campuses planned for Bowling Green and Northern Kentucky. The Rural Physician Leadership Program (RPLP) was designed to leverage a long-term teaching relationship between the UK COM and St. Claire Regional Medical Center, a 159-bed rural hospital created in 1963 as a UK teaching affiliate in Morehead, Kentucky. St. Claire was previously an established site for one-month rural experiences. In 2009, the site was accredited as a two-year clinical rural campus. Our first students arrived in 2010. The mission of the RPLP is "to increase the number of physicians who are trained to provide high-quality health care, who are knowledgeable about community health, and who will address the acute shortage of physicians in the rural areas of the Commonwealth." Located 66 miles from the main campus, we are one of 39 national rural tracks. In a recent study, our program was noted to be the most rural in the nation.

Structure, Governance, and Funding:

The RPLP is directed by an Assistant Dean who is assisted by a part-time (M.D.) curriculum director. Two clinical clerkship coordinators, an admissions assistant and a student affairs assistant complete the staff. The program contracts with the local Area Health Education Center (AHEC) to credential and coordinate faculty. The RPLP budget includes staff salaries, and 10 percent funding for clinical clerkship directors. Funding is provided entirely by the UK College of Medicine through an annual budget.

Student Body:

The RPLP enrolls 10 students per year. To date, 87 students have matriculated into nine classes. Most students (80 percent) are Kentucky residents. The program has also welcomed 18 out-of-state students, many of whom have personal ties and a vested interest in Kentucky. Of particular note, 39 percent of in-state students hail from counties with a poverty rate greater than 25 percent. Over half (52 percent) of enrolled students are women.

Of our 48 graduates, two-thirds (65 percent) have gone into primary care career fields. Students have also matched into a breadth of other specialties, including psychiatry, surgery, and neurosurgery.

Admission to RPLP is currently a separate process driven by the regional campus. All admission decisions are subject to final approval by the main campus. As part of the admissions process, prospective students travel to Morehead to interview with our regional campus Admissions Committee. This committee is comprised of local business persons, faculty, and students. Monthly informational open houses are hosted by the Assistant Dean, current students, and administrative staff to recruit potential students. In these sessions, we discuss the admissions process and regional curriculum in greater detail with interested applicants.

The RPLP also sponsors a week long "admissions boot camp" for college students potentially interested in rural medicine. Students receive feedback about their medical school applications, and learn interview skills and general tips to prepare them for the admissions process.

Curriculum:

Our students spend their first and second years integrated with 126 classmates at the main campus. They participate in a block curriculum that is structured by organ systems. For all small group activities, the RPLP students are placed together and paired with RPLP faculty.

After the second year, students move to Morehead to complete their clinical rotations. The core third-year courses share common syllabi with the main campus. Mandatory lectures from the main campus are live-streamed to RPLP students via teleconference. Students complete rotations in Internal Medicine, Emergency Medicine, OB-GYN, Surgery, Neurology, Psychiatry, and Pediatrics. Family Medicine is structured as a longitudinal experience throughout the entire year. Family Medicine is mostly outpatient, and includes house calls, inpatient, and maternity care elements designed to highlight the versatile role of the rural family physician.

During fourth year, acting internships and an array of other electives are available at our regional campus. Electives are also available at the main campus for more specialized rotations if they are needed for specific residency applications.

Unique Characteristics:

Access to patients is one of the greatest advantages of our regional campus. During the summer of first and second year, students come to Morehead for a two-week personalized clinical experience. During this time, students learn to independently perform and document patient histories as active participants on the clinical care team.

RPLP covers tuition costs for third-year students interested in a year-long course in Healthcare Leadership at Morehead State University. The course has six four-week modules, covering topics such as health insurance models, basic business theories, healthcare ethics, and leadership styles. Students completing the course receive a certificate in health leadership.

A particular strength of our program is the on-site availability of administrative staff at our rural regional campus.

Accomplishments and Challenges:

Our students have regularly occupied leadership positions at the main campus. Two class vice presidents and one class president have come from the RPLP. Two of our graduates have also been selected for prestigious fellowship positions at Stanford University and the Mayo Clinic.

One of our biggest challenges has been finding a rural Neurology experience. The RPLP currently provides housing for students to complete their neurology rotation in Richmond, Kentucky, 60 miles away. Another challenge has been pediatric exposure. The rural Pediatrics rotation is primarily outpatient. To supplement this, the main campus has agreed to provide an inpatient experience for our students.

Many of our clerkships rely on a single physician for clinical exposure. While this fosters a close relationship between faculty and students, when clinicians have time off, teaching is potentially compromised. Finding time for busy rural clinicians to communicate with their main campus counterparts has also been a challenge. Email, phone conversations, and site visits are the primary means of communication. In addition, two annual faculty development events (one in Lexington and one in Morehead) have been organized to encourage communication, collaboration, and networking between sites.

Future Plans:

In the next several years, the RPLP will transition to a four-year program located entirely in Morehead. We plan to use a combination of distance learning and local Morehead State University faculty to teach basic sciences. Students will also train interprofessionally with PA students, Pharmacy residents, DNP students, and PT and Social Work students in our small rural community. We plan to expand our admissions and recruiting resources to maintain our high-quality rural education program.

Additional long-term plans include improving our business and leadership curriculum, developing partnerships with other healthcare facilities to provide more stability for our clinical rotations, and possibly developing a dedicated three-year primary care curriculum.

19. University of Massachusetts Medical School - Baystate

Authors:

- Rebecca D. Blanchard, Ph.D.,
  Senior Director of Educational Affairs and Assistant Dean
  for Education, Associate Professor of Medicine,
  University of Massachusetts Medical School-Baystate

- Kevin T. Hinchey, M.D.,
  Chief Education Officer and Senior Associate Dean
  for Education, Associate Professor of Medicine,
  University of Massachusetts Medical School-Baystate

Regional Campus:

University of Massachusetts Medical School - Baystate
Location: Springfield, Massachusetts

Institution (main campus):

University of Massachusetts Medical School
Location: Worcester, Massachusetts

History and Mission:

As an institution with nationally recognized educators, the only tertiary care referral center in western Massachusetts, and a Level-I trauma center, Baystate Health has been a top teaching site for students and residents across various health professions for over 30 years. Each year, this independent academic medical center hosts approximately 30 third-year medical students for core clinical rotations and over 200 fourth-year students in 45 different electives.

In 2016, Baystate Health and University of Massachusetts Medical School (UMMS) built on the location, mission, and strengths of Baystate Health, naming it the regional campus of *University of Massachusetts Medical School-Baystate* (UMMS-Baystate), and created the Population-based Urban and Rural Community Health (PURCH) track. The PURCH track focuses on care for the underserved, and encourages students to think comprehensively about population health, social determinants of health, disease prevention, and wellness. UMMS-Baystate admits only 25 students per year to the PURCH track to ensure a rich, valuable experience for students and patients.

As the first and only public medical school for the Commonwealth of Massachusetts, UMMS was founded in 1962 on the principle of training high-quality primary care physicians for state residents. UMMS-Baystate embraces this mission, emphasizing patient-centered experiences in urban and rural community health.

While PURCH students participate in most of their core curriculum at the main campus in years one and two, they regularly travel just under 60 miles to UMMS-Baystate for rich, innovative, and immersive experiences which fulfill a portion of their curricular requirements. These courses are taught by UMMS-Baystate in the new educational space designed and built specifically for the students.

Structure, Governance and Funding:

UMMS-Baystate is led by a regional executive dean and a leadership team that includes a Senior Associate Dean for Education, Assistant

Dean for Education, Associate Dean for Research, and Associate Dean for Faculty Affairs. In addition, UMMS-Baystate has an Assistant Dean of Admissions, who oversees the admissions process for the regional campus in collaboration with the main campus.

As a regional campus of the system, UMMS-Baystate faculty participate in the Educational Policy Committee, the main faculty governance committee for the medical school. UMMS-Baystate faculty also serve on curriculum committees for all four years and for their own PURCH curriculum committee.

Student Body:

UMMS-Baystate students participate in their basic science core courses at the main campus in Worcester, Massachusetts. Approximately 19 days per year during their first and second years, UMMS-Baystate students travel to Springfield for their PURCH track courses, immersive experiences in clinical settings, and meetings with PURCH track mentors. In their third and fourth years, UMMS-Baystate students participate in their clinical rotations at the 716-bed Baystate Medical Center, or across the three community hospitals in the Baystate Health System: Baystate Noble Hospital, Baystate Franklin Medical Center, and Baystate Wing Hospital.

UMMS admits 150 students per year. Of these students, approximately 25 will participate in the PURCH track at UMMS-Baystate and 10 students will participate in the UMMS M.D./Ph.D. program. UMMS is a public state university, and for over 50 years, only admitted Massachusetts residents. In 2015, UMMS opened 15 percent of their spots for out-of-state students, enrolling a class that was 54 percent female, 20 percent first-generation college graduates, and 14 percent from groups underrepresented in medicine.

Prospective students must apply to UMMS through the American Medical College Application Service (AMCAS). Once the application is verified by UMMS, the student is sent instructions for completing an online secondary application which includes a supplemental application for the PURCH track.

Only applicants who meet the standards for academic criteria set by the main campus are considered for admission to the UMMS-Baystate PURCH track. If invited to interview, prospective PURCH track students complete a two-day interview, with the first day at the main campus and the second day at UMMS-Baystate. Both UMMS and UMMS-Baystate include multiple mini interviews (MMIs). UMMS-Baystate has a separate admissions committee which recommends students for admission to the UMMS admission committee. Applications are considered on a rolling basis and interviews are conducted September through March.

While not all students applying to UMMS-Baystate PURCH track are seeking to enter primary care, most express an interest in caring for the underserved and express an interest in community health. Many are also from the catchment area of Baystate Health, which includes not only western Massachusetts, but also southern Vermont, eastern New York, and northern Connecticut.

Curriculum:

The PURCH track creates empathetic physicians who are reflective diagnosticians, leaders who can be led, and collaborative team members. These five pillars of empathy, diagnostic skills, collaborative leadership, team-oriented approach, and reflective thinking guide the content of PURCH courses. PURCH students identify opportunities to reform the health care system and care for a diverse group of patients in urban and rural settings. Primary teaching methods for the first and second year courses include small group sessions, interactions with real patients, peer-teaching, and faculty-student mentoring.

PURCH students receive the same curriculum content that is provided to UMMS students at the main campus. There are three main curricular components taught in the first year and all are considerably integrated. These include:

1. **Doctoring and Clinical Skills (DCS):** Small group sessions with students and faculty facilitators promote learning and practicing skills included in the core competencies, such as the medical interview, clinical reasoning, teamwork, and presentation skills. This component includes extensive experience with patients from the community.

2. **Physical Diagnosis (PD):** In this course, students are taught the skills needed to examine patients and formulate a diagnosis. It includes both didactics and hands-on experience, working to overlap organ systems addressed in physical diagnosis sessions with the students' gross anatomy course taught at the main campus. At the Baystate campus, PD sessions are incorporated into the DCS curriculum.

3. **The Longitudinal Preceptorship Program (LPP):** This program places students into a consistent community clinical setting beginning in the first weeks of medical school, providing the opportunity to practice skills taught in small groups or PD sessions, and to interact with patients under the supervision of an assigned faculty physician preceptor at clinical sites within a 30-minute radius of the Baystate campus.

Unique Characteristics:

UMMS-Baystate students have their own Learning Community at the regional campus, named after a local community. The Brightwood Learning Community includes four UMMS-Baystate faculty mentors who provide consistent mentoring for PURCH students throughout all four years.

The community of Springfield is greatly involved with the PURCH track. For example, several community partners have trained as standardized patients to help teach PURCH students.

UMMS-Baystate also has access to the teaching academy of an interprofessional community of educators, called Baystate Education Research and Scholarship of Teaching (BERST) Academy. BERST Academy leads professional development to ensure faculty and preceptors hone their skills as teachers and educators to maintain high quality education in PURCH and a consistent language across all faculty at the Baystate campus. The Academy emphasizes similar pillars as the PURCH track, and produces teachers that inculcate those values.

Future Plans:

UMMS-Baystate is a recent partnership between two institutions with very rich histories. The enthusiasm for the opportunities created by this collaboration benefits UMMS-Baystate students by providing access to two campuses, each with teachers and mentors who care very deeply about their success. Among other future plans for curricular innovation is the development of a Longitudinal Curriculum for PURCH students.

20. University of Minnesota Medical School, Duluth Campus

Authors:

- Paula M. Termuhlen, M.D.,
  Regional Campus Dean, Professor of Surgery (with tenure),
  University of Minnesota Medical School, Duluth Campus

- Alan M. Johns, M.D., M.Ed.,
  Associate Dean for Curriculum and Technology, Assistant
  Professor of Family Medicine and Biobehavioral Health,
  University of Minnesota Medical School, Duluth Campus

Regional Campus:

University of Minnesota Medical School, Duluth Campus
Location: Duluth, Minnesota

Institution (main campus):

University of Minnesota Medical School
Location: Minneapolis, Minnesota

History and Mission:

In 1972, The University of Minnesota Duluth School of Medicine was founded in Duluth, Minnesota as a separate Liaison Committee on Medical Education (LCME) accredited independent unit of the land-grant University of Minnesota, with a curriculum that spanned the first two years of medical school. The initial proposal was a collaborative effort of state and local physicians who not only saw the need for additional physicians in greater Minnesota, but also recognized the value of producing an increased number of family physicians who were uniquely suited to serve in rural communities. Located 150 miles (2 ½ hours by car) from the University of Minnesota, Twin Cities campus, the University of Minnesota Duluth served as the academic home and geographic location for the school. The new school was created through a legislative appropriation as a means to increase the physician workforce in rural Minnesota. After completing the first two years of medical school, it was anticipated that the majority of students would transition to the medical school on the Twin Cities campus since the original curriculum was designed to allow a seamless transfer.

Shortly after the first class was started, the mission was broadened to encourage the development of Native American physicians in recognition of the large American Indian population of Minnesota which was grossly underserved. A number of pipeline programs and initiatives to support American Indian and Alaska Native medical students were created as part of a Center for American Indian and Minority Health (CAIMH), housed on the Duluth Campus. An example is the Native Americans into Medicine (NAM) program that was created in 1973 and continues to host undergraduate students for six weeks in the summer, introducing them to careers in science and medicine. The NAM program also provides mentorship in preparing undergraduate students to apply to medical school and other health professions. Another summer program is the Pre-matriculation Program which allows medical students to come a month early and meet other students in the setting of a mock medical school course. Students practice study skills in a low-stakes format and are introduced to problem-based learning (PBL). It gives students a chance to be leaders when classes start by showing other students how to effectively navigate PBL sessions and lectures. In honor of our mission to serve Native people, Native American heritage is celebrated on our campus with ceremonial activities, such as smudging and drumming, at key medical school events like the White Coat Ceremony and Graduation.

In 2002, the LCME required that all accredited medical schools have a full curriculum leading to the terminal degree. A decision was made by the University of Minnesota, Duluth School of Medicine to combine with the University of Minnesota Medical School and become a regional campus. Thus, it was renamed as the University of Minnesota Medical School, Duluth Campus on July 1, 2003. The mission of serving rural and Native American communities by increasing physician workforce was preserved and expanded.

The University of Minnesota Medical School was founded in 1888 as the College of Medicine and Surgery. It is widely known for a variety of ground-breaking work including the first bone marrow transplant, the first intestinal transplant, and the first successful open-heart surgery. Since 1970, it has been part of a large Academic Health Center (AHC) with six professional schools in Medicine, Pharmacy, Nursing, Public Health, Dentistry, and Veterinary Medicine. The College of Pharmacy also has a regional campus located in Duluth. The National Center for Interprofessional Education and Practice resides within the AHC and provides a platform for interprofessional learning and development among the students and faculty. The University of Minnesota Medical School graduates 230 students annually with one-quarter of them beginning their studies on the Duluth Campus.

Among Regional Medical Campuses, the Duluth Campus is unique in that the majority of faculty are scientists who conduct basic science research or engage in community-based participatory research. The Duluth Campus location at the University of Minnesota Duluth provides opportunities to engage with undergraduates to foster careers in science and medicine. The medical school campus participates in the

Integrated Biological Sciences program with the Department of Biology and the regional campus of the College of Pharmacy to train graduate students in scientific disciplines leading to masters and doctoral degrees. The faculty are also able to participate in the Graduate Studies programs of the University of Minnesota Twin Cities.

Beyond producing a physician workforce for rural and Native American communities, the Duluth Campus of the University of Minnesota Medical School is a recognized expert in health disparity research, being noted as one of the top four for work with Native peoples by the National Institutes of Health. A state-legislated Medical Discovery Team resides on the Duluth Campus with a focus on health equity in Native American and Rural populations. In addition, the campus has recently received a large gift to support a Center of Excellence in Native American Health Research and Education.

Nationally, the University of Minnesota Medical School, Duluth Campus has been a leader in the AAMC Group on Regional Medical Campuses with two faculty serving consecutively as members of the GRMC Steering Committee. In service to regional campuses across North America and in partnership with the University of Minnesota Libraries, the Duluth Campus sponsors the *Journal of Regional Medical Campuses.* Launched in 2017, this online, open-access journal is designed to provide a place to share the scholarship found on Regional Medical Campuses in the United States and Canada.

Structure, Governance and Funding:

The Duluth Campus is led by a Regional Campus Dean who reports directly to the Dean of the Medical School and is part of the Medical School senior leadership team. Campus-based associate deans for curriculum and technology, student affairs and admissions, rural health, and research provide administrative infrastructure. The Duluth Campus has staff level support in the form of an administrative center with a director that mirrors the units found on the Twin Cities Campus. Faculty of the Duluth Campus participate as full members of the Medical School. Specific positions on key Medical School and University Committees, such as Promotion and Tenure, Faculty Advisory Council, and Faculty Consultative Committee must be filled by Duluth Campus faculty.

The campus receives all of the tuition monies from its students. Faculty who are funded-investigators also help to support salary and research operations. The campus receives a significant portion of direct and indirect federal and foundation research dollars awarded to successful investigators. In addition, there are special legislative funds related to research and rural education that are part of campus revenue. The Duluth Campus has its own development officer who raises funds for scholarships and research.

Student Body:

Sixty students are recruited annually for a total of 120 students on the campus. One hundred and seventy students matriculate on the Twin Cities campus each year. After completing the first two years on the Duluth Campus, students are merged with their Twin Cities Campus peers and graduate as a single class.

Prospective students may apply to both the Twin Cities and the Duluth campuses. Using a holistic review process, the Duluth Campus specifically seeks to admit students who are from rural Minnesota communities with an interest in Family Medicine or who wish to serve Native American people. Eighty percent of the admitted students come from communities with populations of 20,000 or less. One-third meet AMCAS definitions of disadvantaged socioeconomic status. On average, 10 percent of the class is Native American. In partnership with the University of Minnesota Duluth, a small cohort of students is admitted annually (up to five) who are able to receive their bachelor's degree after completing the first year of medical school. Ninety percent of students are from Minnesota. The only out-of-state students are those who are American Indian or Alaska Native. Approximately 50 percent of students choose Family Medicine as a career.

After completing the first two years of school on the Duluth Campus, students are able to participate in the dual degree programs offered by the University of Minnesota Medical School including the M.D.-Ph.D., the M.D.-MPH, M.D.-MBA and M.D.-JD programs, if they desire.

Curriculum:

The Duluth Campus curriculum spans 24 months with a primary focus on the foundational sciences delivered in an integrated system format. Approximately one-half of the material is delivered in a small group, active learning format. Most of the students attend class, which adds to the cohesiveness of the groups. Embedded within the first two years is a rural curriculum including:

- Introduction to Rural Family Medicine (required Year One)
- Rural Academy of Leadership (elective)
- Family Medicine OB Longitudinal Course (elective)
- Family Medicine Preceptorship (Duluth-based; required)
- Rural Medical Scholars Program (required; students spend five one-week sessions at the same rural site in Minnesota with a Family Medicine physician over the course of both years)

- Summer Internship in Medicine (elective open to both campuses that allows students to shadow a rural physician of any specialty in Minnesota)

In addition to the offerings to enhance understanding of rural practice, there is a nationally-recognized, required course that introduces students to Native American health and culture.

In years three and four, students are able to participate in one of three tracks:

- The Rural Physician Associate Program (RPAP) is one of the original longitudinal integrated clerkships (LIC). After having a core internal medicine experience, students spend the remainder of year three in a rural setting. Medical School faculty enhance the learning experiences by flying and driving to the sites located throughout the state to participate in case conferences and to deliver clinical lectures.

- Traditional discipline-based experiences in the Twin Cities or in Duluth

- Urban, Suburban, and Veterans Administration Hospital LICs where students spend nine months of year three in a specific setting.

Unique Characteristics:

The unique characteristics of the Duluth Campus are found within its mission. Students are specifically recruited from rural communities and Native American communities and return to practice in these settings at a rate much higher than national averages. The faculty cohort on the

Duluth Campus reflects the diversity of its student body. Known as a best practice within the Medical School, six of its 42 faculty are Native persons and another five represent other under-represented groups in science and medicine. Fifty percent of the faculty and campus leadership are women.

Accomplishments and Challenges:

In 2017, the University of Minnesota Medical School was ranked Number 1 in graduates who pursue Family Medicine as a career and Number 2 in graduating American Indian and Alaska Native physicians. This in large part is due to the contributions of the Duluth Campus. Approximately 50 percent of graduates who start on the Duluth Campus pursue Family Medicine. Retention of graduates is robust with almost two-thirds remaining in the state of Minnesota for practice. Service to rural Minnesota remains high with 44 percent of graduates practicing in communities of 25,000 or less.

The challenges of the Duluth Campus are similar to other campuses. Ongoing work to ensure financial sustainability continues. Competition from other learners for preceptor sites and time is keen. However, many of the preceptors are alumni who remain loyal to the University of Minnesota and its missions.

Future Plans:

Future plans for the University of Minnesota Medical School, Duluth Campus include expanding the class size to 70 per year and creating tracks which allow for students to complete all four years in Duluth or a rural setting. Additional areas of focused research programs in alignment with the missions are being considered.

21. University of South Dakota Sanford School of Medicine

Authors:

- Mark Beard, M.D., MHA,
  Assistant Dean of Medical Student Education,
  Associate Professor, Department of Family Medicine,
  University of South Dakota Sanford School of Medicine,
  Sioux Falls Campus

- Shane Schellpfeffer, Ed.D.,
  Director of Evaluation and Assessment,
  Assistant Professor, Department of Neurosciences,
  University of South Dakota Sanford School of Medicine,
  Sioux Falls Campus

Regional Campus:

University of South Dakota Sanford School of Medicine
Location: State of South Dakota

Institution (main campus):

University of South Dakota Sanford School of Medicine
Location: State of South Dakota

History and Mission:

The University of South Dakota (USD), the state's flagship university, was founded in 1862 and is the state's oldest university. Accredited by the North Central Association of Colleges and Schools since 1913, USD is a comprehensive, doctorate-granting institution with a liberal arts undergraduate emphasis.

The University of South Dakota, Sanford School of Medicine (SSOM) is one medical school, with multiple regional campuses spread throughout the State of South Dakota. The College of Medicine was organized in 1907 and existed initially as a two-year medical school. In 1974, the South Dakota Legislature authorized a complete four-year degree-granting program of medical education oriented towards primary care. Accreditation was granted by the LCME in 1975, and the school graduated its first M.D. class in 1977. In 2005, the school was renamed the University of South Dakota Sanford School of Medicine in recognition of a $20 million endowment from South Dakota philanthropist, T. Denny Sanford.

The SSOM is a community-based medical school with a basic science campus in Vermillion, and three clinical campuses located in Sioux Falls (two locations), Rapid City, and Yankton. A limited number of students complete their primary clinical year in seven rural communities as part of the Frontier and Rural Medicine (FARM) program. The main administrative offices for the medical school are located in Sioux Falls. (See Section 3 under South Dakota Sanford School of Medicine for a map and driving distances between campuses).

The mission of the SSOM is to provide the opportunity for South Dakota residents to receive a quality, broad-based medical education with an emphasis on family medicine, and to provide students and the people of South Dakota excellence in education, research, and service.

Structure, Governance and Funding:

The governance of the SSOM is central and distributed. The Vice President of Health Affairs/SSOM Dean is responsible for all administration of the medical school. The Dean is the chief academic officer who oversees the medical education program. The majority of the curriculum management is delegated to the Dean of Medical Student Education. The principal academic officers (campus deans) at each clinical campus and the director of the FARM program report to the SSOM Dean.

As a public community-based medical school, the SSOM relies on state appropriations, tuition and fees to support its academic mission. State appropriations account for roughly one-third of operating revenues. These appropriations were recently increased to fund class expansion and the implementation of the FARM program. Tuition and fees, grants and contracts, revenue, gifts, and endowments make up the remainder of supporting funds. Hospital system revenue also provides support by funding graduate medical education.

Student Body:

The SSOM admits 67 categorical four-year M.D. students, two INMED (Indians in Medicine) students, and two M.D./Ph.D. students annually, for a total entering class size of 71 students. The SSOM has expanded its entering class by one-third over the last decade. The school also offers a doctor of philosophy degree in Basic Biomedical Sciences.

The medical school is known for its emphasis on family medicine and rural medicine. Over 75 percent of the students come from South Dakota, with 66 different high schools represented. Approximately 30 percent of students are graduates of South Dakota high schools in towns with populations less than 10,000.

Curriculum:

The SSOM Yankton Model Ambulatory Program has been at the forefront of curriculum reform as a Longitudinal Integrated Clerkship (LIC) since 1991. As a result of the success of the Yankton model, the SSOM effected a broad curriculum revision in 2013 with the introduction of a novel Three Pillar Curriculum. Pillar One includes a shorter pre-clerkship curriculum of integrated organ-system blocks. Pillar Two, the primary clinical year, uses the LIC model at all campuses and sites. Residency preparation experiences and electives comprise Pillar Three.

The curriculum begins with three semesters of basic biomedical science education at the Vermillion campus. During the first year, students also select one of three clinical sites — Sioux Falls (two locations), Rapid City, or Yankton — where they will finish the final two pillars of medical school (see below). A small number of students are selected for the FARM program as well. Students who enter the FARM program return to one of the three clinical sites for their final pillar of training. During the final pillar, students may take clinical rotations at any of the four clinical campuses due to the flexibility in scheduling.

During Pillar Two, students average a half day per week in each of the seven major disciplines to gain clinical competence across multiple disciplines. Students acquire experience by managing problem-focused encounters and selecting appropriate treatment plans. Each campus adheres to the guiding SSOM competencies and educational requirements, with some variability between the campuses based on local needs.

Unique Characteristics:

The most unique characteristic of the SSOM is the implementation of competency-based education. The competencies form the guiding principles of the education program, and serve as stand-alone courses in Pillar Two. Student performance is assessed for all competencies using a letter grade supplemented by narrative comments. Another unique feature of the Pillar 2 curriculum are the LIC and FARM program Coordinating Committees. The Coyote Clinic, a free student-run clinic based in Sioux Falls, is managed by Pillar Two students. The Coyote Clinic offers free healthcare to uninsured patients and provides learning opportunities to medical students across all pillars of the curriculum. A week-long cultural immersion experience is another unique curricular feature. During this week, students study cultural diversity and provide community service at different sites among various cultures across the State of South Dakota.

Accomplishments and Challenges:

In 2013, the Yankton campus received the Shining Star of Education Innovation award from the Association of American Medical Colleges (AAMC) for the Yankton Model Ambulatory Program. Based on the successful community engagement of the SSOM's regional clinical campuses, the SSOM was also honored by the 2017 Spencer Foreman Award for Outstanding Community Service presented by the AAMC.

With the implementation of a LIC model across all campuses, challenges to ensure comparability across all campuses in the curriculum were quickly identified. To address this challenge, curriculum monitoring and student assessment are centrally facilitated by the Office of Medical Education to provide adequate oversight.

Future Plans:

Currently, the SSOM is refining and enhancing its Pillar Three curriculum. Efforts to create clinical competency committees (like those in Pillar Two) are being considered to provide more oversight of student progress. Additional consideration is being given to determine how best to enhance residency preparation at the end of Pillar Three. Ongoing innovations and continued development of current programs will allow the school to continue to grow with a comparable curriculum that is shared across regional campuses in the State of South Dakota.

22. University of South Florida-Lehigh Valley

Authors:

- Margaret A. Hadinger, Ed.D., MS,
  Director of Medical Education,
  Affiliate Assistant Professor of Medicine,
  Lehigh Valley Health Network, Department of Education,
  University of South Florida Morsani College of Medicine

- Jasmine I. Kashkoush, SELECT Class of 2019,
  University of South Florida Morsani College of Medicine

Regional Campus:

University of South Florida-Lehigh Valley
Location: Allentown, Pennsylvania

Institution (main campus):

University of South Florida HEALTH,
Morsani College of Medicine
Location: Tampa, Florida

History and Mission:

Since 1965, the University of South Florida (USF) College of Medicine has transformed into a major academic medical center known for its innovative curriculum with an emphasis on improving health through interprofessional education, research, and clinical activities. USF Health is a partnership between the Colleges of Nursing, Pharmacy, Public Health, School of Physical Therapy and Rehabilitative Sciences, and the Morsani College of Medicine (MCOM). USF MCOM[1], which enrolled its charter class in 1971, awards doctorates in Medicine (M.D.), in addition to Ph.D., DPT, and MS degrees. USF MCOM is located on the main campus of USF in Tampa, Florida.

Lehigh Valley Health Network's (LVHN) legacy of patient-centered care began with the opening of The Allentown Hospital in 1899. Today, LVHN has transformed into one of the nation's most respected health networks, offering care in 95 clinical specialties at eight hospital campuses. Consistent with the Network's vision to continue as a "premier academic community health system," LVHN has a long history of both undergraduate and graduate medical education.

USF MCOM and LVHN affiliated in 2009 with the goal of transforming medical education leadership training. The partnership created a regional branch campus of USF MCOM located in Allentown, PA, known as USF-Lehigh Valley. Simultaneously, the partnership created the SELECT program, with SELECT representing the principles of Scholarly Excellence, Leadership Experiences, and Collaborative Training.

USF MCOM, including the USF-Lehigh Valley regional campus, was awarded full accreditation by the Liaison Committee on Medical Education (LCME) in 2015, with its next review scheduled for 2022-2023. The SELECT program, with years three and four housed at USF-Lehigh Valley, received approval by the Pennsylvania Department of

---

1   The USF College of Medicine was re-named the USF Health Morsani College of Medicine in 2011.

Education in 2010. The first class of SELECT matriculated in 2011 and graduated in 2015.

Structure, Governance, and Funding:

The USF-Lehigh Valley campus is led by the Associate Dean of Educational Affairs, who also serves as LVHN's Chief Academic Officer. The Associate Dean has a dual-report to USF MCOM's Vice Dean for Education, as well as LVHN's Chief Medical Officer. The Associate Dean is assisted by the Assistant Dean for Student Affairs, who has a dual-report to the regional campus Associate Dean as well as to USF MCOM's Associate Dean for Student Affairs in Tampa.

The regional campus Deans are supported by LVHN's Department of Education, namely a Director of Medical Education, Student Affairs Specialists, Faculty Affairs Coordinator, Curriculum Specialist, Technology Specialists, and Simulation Experts, with further support from Information Services, Security, and Library Services.

Positions that directly support SELECT are funded via USF MCOM tuition revenue and student fees.

Student Body:

SELECT students represent a diverse mix of Pennsylvania, Florida, and out-of-state residents. Students are selected via USF MCOM's holistic review process, after choosing to be considered for either the Core program, the SELECT program, or both. Applicants undergo a Behavioral Event Interview (BEI) with one to two faculty using a scoring rubric focused on specific emotional intelligence competencies identified as critical to the development of medical leadership.

Once matriculated, SELECT students complete pre-clinical years one and two at USF-Tampa, alongside their peers in the Core M.D. parallel curriculum. Differentiating SELECT, during the period between the end of their second year and the beginning of their third year, students transition to USF-Lehigh Valley, where they complete their third year. In their fourth year, SELECT students complete five months at USF-Lehigh Valley, and can elect to complete the remainder of their fourth year electives at either the Lehigh Valley or Tampa campuses, or at any approved host site.

Students may participate in Match Day ceremonies in either Pennsylvania or Florida. All USF MCOM students commence in Tampa. To date[2] the Match has yielded:

- 100 percent match rate for 153 graduates
- 27 PA matches
- 30 FL matches
- 15 LVHN matches
- 52 primary care matches

Curriculum:

SELECT students complete third-year clerkships, including a longitudinal Primary Care clerkship and 12-week integrated clerkships in Women's Health and Pediatrics, Surgical Care, Neurology-Psychiatry, and Adult Medicine. The inclusion of a longitudinal Primary Care

---

2   For the Classes of 2015, 2016, 2017, and 2018.

clerkship — in comparison to the block Primary Care clerkship required of the Core program students — provides SELECT students an opportunity to develop relationships with faculty and patients across many months. While on clerkships, students alternate between three weeks of inpatient and three weeks of ambulatory experience, ensuring that students experience both inpatient and ambulatory medicine in nearly equal proportions.

The SELECT four-year curriculum augments the Core medical curriculum with additional coursework and experiences centered on leadership development, health systems, and values-based, patient-centered care. The leadership curriculum is founded on principles of emotional intelligence including: self-awareness, self-management, social awareness, and relationship management.

SELECT students participate in six required courses spanning their four years. Beginning with SELECT Prologues in years one and two, students complete the required longitudinal SELECT 1 and 2 courses, in additional to integrated basic science coursework. Between years one and two, SELECT students complete a required Summer Immersion course, in which students are required to complete a scholarly work related to one of the three SELECT domains. After transitioning to USF-Lehigh Valley, students complete the longitudinal SELECT 3 course and begin the longitudinal Capstone research course. In year four, students complete SELECT 4 — consisting of a two-week Prologue introductory session, asynchronous learning/assignments, and culminating in a one-week Epilogue session — and also complete their required Capstone research project.

Unique Characteristics:

SELECT differs from the Core program in that students physically transition to PA. In addition, they participate in a four-year longitudinal SELECT curriculum focused on the domains of leadership, health systems, and values based patient centered care. The Primary Care and the outpatient Pediatric, Internal Medicine, and Family Medicine experiences provide SELECT students with additional clinical exposure and opportunities to foster relationships with faculty and patients.

Furthermore, SELECT provides professional development coaching for students by grouping six to 10 students with two physician-coaches, one based at USF-Tampa and the other at USF-Lehigh Valley. Coaches form bonds with students as they promote personal and professional growth over the four years. Also, SELECT allows more accessibility of faculty, due to a lower student to faculty ratio.

While at the USF-Lehigh Valley campus, SELECT students have the opportunity to volunteer with Lehigh Valley agencies, including Valley Youth House and LVHN's Street Medicine Program. Students participate in student organizations including Women in Medicine, Art, and Medicine, and various specialty-related interest groups.

SELECT graduates earn an M.D. degree, plus a graduate certificate in Scholarly Excellence, Leadership Experiences, and Collaborative Training.

Accomplishments and Challenges:

Elements that have proven critical to the success of the partnership of USF MCOM and LVHN include: strong leadership support, aligned cultures and shared clarity of purpose/goals, shared accountability, an all-in mentality, and a focus on effective change management and relationship building.

In any partnership, and in particular with partnerships spanning more than 1,000 miles, communication is key. Over the first decade, a focus has been on building and maintaining relationships through opening clear channels for communication. The partnership has negotiated a number of important challenges including creating shared understanding across corporate/clinical and academic cultures and integrating the inherent differences in faculty compensation models.

Future Plans:

Future plans for SELECT including offering a Master's level degree to graduates. Currently SELECT students rotate at LVHN's three primary hospitals in addition to ambulatory experiences. As LVHN continues to merge with other regional hospitals, student experiences may extend further into an ever-widening sphere of PA counties.

23. University of Washington School of Medicine, Spokane Campus

Authors:

- John McCarthy, M.D.,
  Assistant Dean for Rural Programs,
  Clinical Professor of Family Medicine,
  University of Washington School of Medicine, Gonzaga Campus

- Darryl Potyk, M.D., FACP,
  Associate Dean for Eastern Washington,
  Chief of Medical Education for UW School of Medicine-
  Gonzaga University Regional Health Partnership,
  Clinical Associate Professor of Medicine,
  University of Washington School of Medicine, Gonzaga Campus

Regional Campus:

University of Washington School of Medicine,
Gonzaga Campus
Location: Spokane, Washington

Institution:

University of Washington School of Medicine
Location: Seattle, Washington

History and Mission:

In the early 1970s, the University of Washington took on a bold challenge to train and prepare physicians to care for patients and communities throughout the WAMI states, Washington, Alaska, Montana, and Idaho (with Wyoming joining in 1996). Today, this regional medical education program known as WWAMI (an acronym representing the states it serves) continues as an innovative force in medical education.

The WWAMI program has served as a model for the creation of regional medical campuses, while generating a workforce for our five state region where 20 percent of the population lives in rural and underserved communities. The majority of students training in the WWAMI program continue to practice medicine within the five-state region with over half choosing primary care careers.

Each state participating in WWAMI works with the University of Washington School of Medicine (UWSOM) to educate a specified number of medical students from their state. In the WWAMI model, UWSOM partners with a local university to deliver the three-term foundations curriculum (i.e. basic sciences phase). Sites that offer the foundations and clinical curriculum in the same location include Bozeman, Montana, Anchorage, Alaska and Spokane, Washington. Wyoming and Idaho have foundations and clinical experiences in separate locations. This chapter will focus on the Spokane regional campus because it has the largest number of students outside of the central Seattle campus.

The Spokane campus is within the same state as the main campus, although located 300 miles to the east, and hosts 60 students per year. This is the largest cohort outside of the Seattle campus, which is home to 100 students. The Spokane campus is unique in that it represents the first public-private partnership with Gonzaga University. All Regional

Medical Campuses deliver a refreshed curriculum that emphasizes small-group, case-based active learning which was piloted and refined in Spokane. The WWAMI campuses all employ a rapid-cycle continuous quality improvement model to ensure ongoing curriculum refinement, while encouraging educational innovation.

Structure, Governance and Funding:

Spokane has an Associate Dean overseeing all activities. There is an Assistant Dean overseeing the Foundations curriculum delivery and two Assistant Clinical Deans overseeing clinical clerkships in Spokane proper and in Eastern Washington. The majority of the foundational curriculum is delivered by primary care physicians. Curriculum delivery is facilitated by 10 physician guides (each 0.5 FTE), a full-time anatomist (1.0 FTE) supplemented with 1.5 FTE of basic scientists from our partner institution, Gonzaga University. Students are assigned a local physician who serves as a college mentor that facilitates delivery of Fundamentals of Clinical Medicine (FCM), teaching skills such as history taking and physical exams. This mentor also serves as an advisor over the student's four-year medical school career. With a "one to five" ratio, there are 12 college mentors each at 0.25 FTE. The Spokane campus has a combined budget for the Foundations and Clinical curriculum. Staffing allocations, additional study sessions and extracurricular offerings are controlled locally, whereas the majority of the curriculum emanates from the Seattle campus.

Student Body:

In accordance with the WWAMI model, each state pays for the education of its own students and virtually all of students at the Spokane campus are Washington state residents. Washington residents have the option of applying to the Seattle campus, the Spokane Campus or may designate no preference. The Spokane campus offers a smaller class size (60 vs 100) in a medium-sized city (population estimate of 400,000 people) which appeals to many applicants and students. Grade point averages and MCAT scores are similar at the Spokane and at the main campus. The vast majority of students on the Spokane campus designated this site as their preference.

Curriculum:

The Foundations Phase of the curriculum has been shortened from two years to 18 months and is a highly integrated case-based curriculum grounded in active small-group learning. Students receive a Pass/Fail grade with an emphasis on team-based and cooperative learning. The WWAMI campuses are committed to congruence in curriculum delivery and testing. Foundations is followed by two distinct clinical phases; a 12-month Patient Care Phase (required clerkships) and a 15-month Career Explore and Focus Phase (4 required clerkships, plus electives). Students are offered flexible options to best meet their learning styles. For the clinical phases, students may opt for the "Spokane Track", in which most of their clinical experiences are done in and around the Spokane Community. Alternatively, students can do their clinical clerkships in a variety of sites throughout the five-state region where the student will have a rich array of clinical experiences, mentored by community-based clinical faculty volunteering to educate the next generation of physicians. In addition to these traditional block-based models, students may choose to participate in longitudinally integrated clerkships in several settings across the region, as noted below.

- WWAMI Rural Integrated Training Experience (WRITE): A five-month experience in a rural setting.

- Targeted Rural Underserved Track (TRUST): A longitudinal experience within a rural community over a student's entire medical school career. The student becomes integrated within the community, completes WRITE, participates in summer research, and returns regularly to learn about and work in the community.

- Olympia LIC: This year-long Longitudinal Integrated Clerkship spans the Patient Care Phase and part of the Explore and Focus Phase. This experience is offered in the state capital, which is a medium-sized city.

Unique Characteristics:

- The Spokane campus offers a mid-sized class in a mid-sized community where students have the opportunity to work with community-based preceptors and gain exposure to local residency programs. Spokane is an urban tertiary care referral center, but is surrounded by rural communities, so students have a rich variety of clinical experiences.

- The Foundations curriculum is delivered largely by generalist physicians who teach to clinical scenarios. These physicians are practicing clinicians and physician educators.

Within the Foundations and Clinical phases of education, Spokane students are also exposed to a number of Humanities programs that utilize the arts to emphasize professionalism, physical exam skills, reflection, and resilience.

- Beginning in Fall 2018, students may participate in a leadership program lead by local faculty in conjunction with Gonzaga University Organizational Leadership Faculty. Completion of the four-year curriculum will lead to special recognition upon graduation.

- The Spokane campus has an active student-led service-learning program with a variety of programs in which students can participate. These include serving homeless populations, a pipeline group supporting underserved youth (through tutoring and a walking school bus program, and Health Equity Circle [to participate in community organizing activities]).

- We provide many opportunities for collaborative and interprofessional learning. Examples include working with the Gonzaga University Nursing School (ARNP, CRNA, BS programs) and the Gonzaga University Law School, where the medical students have started a medical-legal interest group. In addition, the UWSOM has a Physician Assistant program on campus, as well as an innovative dental program (RIDE: Rural Initiatives in Dental Education), which places dental students in our community. Thus, there are ample interprofessional educational opportunities in Spokane.

Accomplishments and Challenges:

The UWSOM-Spokane campus offers an ideal environment for modern medical education. The regional campuses within our system are places of innovation and the Spokane campus is no different. Together with our regional campuses we led the way by initiating and piloting a newly revised curriculum, as well as the rapid cycle improvement process. The clinical training options are diverse so that students can customize their experience to their needs (i.e. track, LIC, and block curricula throughout the five-state region). Our rural programs (i.e. TRUST/WRITE) and our Humanities programs have been nationally recognized. Continuing to increase the number of clinical training sites in our area is a challenge, given the increasing number of health care learners in the community since a second Spokane medical school opened in 2017. Nevertheless, we have developed a regional campus and community committed to medical education as an effective means to address the diverse needs of our region.

24. Washington State University, Elson S. Floyd College of Medicine

Authors:

- Ralitsa Akins, M.D., Ph.D.,
  Associate Dean of Faculty Affairs, Professor,
  Department of Medical Education and Clinical Sciences,
  Washington State University, Elson S. Floyd College of Medicine

- Hannah Winters MS I;
  *Washington State University, Elson S. Floyd College of Medicine,
  Tri-Cities Campus*

Regional Campus:

Washington State University,
Elson S. Floyd College of Medicine
Locations: Four Regional Clinical Campuses: Everett,
Vancouver, Tri-Cities (Richland) and Spokane, Washington

Institution (main campus):

Washington State University Health Sciences Campus
in Spokane, Elson S. Floyd College of Medicine
Location: Spokane, Washington

History and Mission:

Washington State University is the home of 11 colleges, one of which is the College of Medicine. The main university seat is in Pullman, Washington, with program locations in Spokane, Tri-Cities, Vancouver, Everett, multiple Extension County Offices throughout the state, additional locations for Research and Extension Centers, and online programs offered through the Global Campus. The Spokane Campus is known as the Health Sciences Campus, hosting the College of Medicine (COM), College of Nursing, College of Pharmacy, and many research labs. Therefore, the WSU College of Medicine is located on the WSU Spokane Campus, yet Spokane is the main seat for the COM programs. These programs include Medicine, Speech and Hearing, Nutrition and Exercise Physiology, and graduate Biomedical research. The medical program is delivered on four campuses — Spokane, Everett, Vancouver, and Tri-cities, which are geographically located throughout the State of Washington — two in the North, two in the South, two in the East, and two in the West. All four COM campus locations are considered equal, in the sense that at each of the four locations clinical experiences are provided to one-quarter of the student class, using the same curriculum, student services access, and central oversight. At the same time, the majority of pre-clerkship classes are taught on the Spokane campus, so that campus has a dual existence as the main COM seat, and as a clinical campus location.

The WSU COM is named after the late WSU President Elson S. Floyd, whose tireless work led to the abolishment of a state law dating back to 1917, allowing only the University of Washington to operate a medical school in the State of Washington. On April 1, 2015, the WSU Medical School authorizing bill was signed, and the Elson S. Floyd College of Medicine achieved Preliminary Accreditation from LCME in October 2016.

The College's vision is, "Inspiring people to solve problems in challenging health care environments." Its mission is to be:

> "a unique resource for the State of Washington, converging on solutions to the health care triple aim of improving the patient experience of care, keeping populations healthy, and decreasing the cost of care, all while improving the work life of health care providers. Through a culture based on valuing the individual, we will be resourceful, agile, inventive, and generous in serving the people of the state and beyond, to develop healthier populations through research, innovation, inter-professional education, and patient-centered care."

The College is a community-based medical school and started with the simultaneous development of its four regional campuses. Multiple affiliations with clinical partners at all locations are ensuring the richness of the student clinical experiences. The class size is 60 students. The class is divided into four groups, called "Learning Communities," and each Learning Community of 15 students has a "home" in one of the four regional campuses. During the pre-clerkship phase, each student visits his/her home campus six times, for one week at a time, and during the third and fourth years, students will complete their Longitudinal Integrated Clerkships and most of the electives at the assigned campus. The four campuses are very young, and function under the vision and mission of the COM, without formulating their own missions. The curriculum and student activities are the same on each campus, with central oversight from Spokane.

While the Spokane regional campus is co-located in the same city as the College's main campus, Vancouver is 360 miles southwest and Everett is 310 miles west (about a six-hour drive to each), and Tri-cities is located

140 miles south (about a two-hour drive). Vancouver and Everett are most easily accessed through short, one-hour flights to Seattle, Washington, and Portland, Oregon, respectively, and a short drive from the airport to the campus. Video-conferencing is a preferred method for communications between the campuses and allows meaningful meeting participation. Video options such as Skype for Business, Zoom, and RealPresence, as well as Slack channels, are used to streamline communications.

The Inaugural Class:

The WSU Elson S. Floyd College of Medicine's inaugural class included Washington State residents (57/60 students, 95 percent of the class), and three students who had strong ties to the state, such as being born in Washington, having had a childhood address in Washington, graduating from a high school in the state, and/or having a parent or legal guardian who were living in the state at the time of application. 33 percent of the students in the first class came from a low socio-economic status, and 18 percent were first-generation college graduates. Students brought a wide range of undergraduate experiences with a diverse range of science degrees, such as pre-med/biology, neuroscience, and human physiology. Students with degrees in the arts and humanities (e.g., philosophy, history, peace studies) brought valuable insights and perspectives to create a well-rounded class dynamic.

Over 700 applications were submitted in the short span of 27 days, the period between the preliminary accreditation approval and the application deadline. At the time of application, prospective students were asked to select a desired campus assignment. To help decision-making, the school offered an opportunity for an additional visit in the spring for admitted students, called "Second Look", that provided further information about the school and the local area. The admission requirements for Washington residency or proof of strong ties with the state will continue to apply for future applicants. The intent is to engage students who will want to return to their underserved rural or urban communities to practice medicine.

How the Students Experience the Curriculum:

Students experience the same curriculum organization and content, notwithstanding their campus allocation. As one student described it,

> "The basic science courses are taught alongside classes exploring the less definable, yet equally indispensable, aspects of becoming a doctor. This includes discussing, learning, and training in the art and practice of medicine, as well as digging into how to critically evaluate the plethora, and ever-increasing amount of scientific knowledge in an evidence-based medicine environment."

Content comprehension is tested weekly, and an integrated case-based learning approach is utilized. Students, divided into small groups, begin each week with a new clinical case, knowledge gaps are addressed during the week, and the experience culminates with presentations of differential diagnoses and an interactive session with a master clinician.

Unique Features:

The Elson S. Floyd students will graduate with a medical degree and a Certificate in Leadership. The leadership program aims to address the changing landscape of the medical field, to prepare them to become participants and leaders in interprofessional teams that will function best when led well. The demands placed on individuals in medical careers point to the need for intentional personal development in areas such as emotional intelligence and effective communication, topics that the leadership courses address.

The students will experience patient continuity through the planned Longitudinal Integrated Clerkship anchored in each of the four clinical campuses. The students will follow their own panel of patients over the long-term longevity of the clerkship and will get a chance to witness and support the full range of the patients' experiences.

A unique feature of the Elson S. Floyd program is the intentional focus on interprofessional education. Multiple health-professions programs are offered on campus, such as Speech and Hearing, Nutrition and Exercise Physiology, Nursing, and Pharmacy to name only a few. This naturally fosters opportunities to begin relationship-building with other health professionals.

Another unique feature of the medical school is the development of the Technology Incubator, where students can explore and contribute to how modern technology is integrated into innovative advancements in medicine. The students also are offered an opportunity to personally experience P4 medicine and its components, including, but not limited to genetic testing. From the students' perspective, there are many "firsts" that the inaugural class has already experienced. Additionally, many more exciting "firsts" will be experienced by this and future classes of resourceful, agile, inventive, and generous students. These motivated learners will fulfill the school's mission through research, innovation, an interprofessional focus, and patient-centered care.

25. West Virginia University School of Medicine, Eastern Division

Authors:

- Rosemarie Cannarella Lorenzetti M.D., MPH,
  Professor of Family Medicine, Associate Dean of Faculty
  Affairs, Associate Dean of Student Services,
  WVU Eastern Campus

- K.C. Nau M.D.,
  Professor Emeritus- Department of Family Medicine,
  Previous Dean and Associate VP of *WVU Eastern Campus*
  (retired July 2017)

- Eleanor Smith M.D.,
  Assistant Professor of Pediatrics,
  Pediatric Faculty lead for the Rural Family Medicine residency,
  Former *Eastern Division* Student

Regional Campus:

West Virginia University School of Medicine, Eastern Campus
Location: Martinsburg, West Virginia

Institution (main campus):

West Virginia University School of Medicine
Location: Morgantown, West Virginia

History and Mission:

West Virginia University School of Medicine (WVU-SOM) – Eastern Campus Division was created in 2002, with a mission to provide medical education and to fulfill the health care needs of citizens in the Eastern Panhandle. It was the University's second branch campus, and was established in the Eastern Panhandle, one of the state's highest population growth areas. It was also one of the first U.S. medical campuses founded with a Longitudinal Integrated Curriculum (LIC) model, designed to best use local physician resources. The formal educational and administrative building for the campus is in Martinsburg, West Virginia, located 150 miles east of the main campus in Morgantown. The "clinical education campus" is spread out over three Eastern Panhandle counties. Accreditation was awarded in 2004, and the LIC model is still in use today.

When the Eastern Campus was formed in 2002, the academic structure for Faculty Development and Promotion and Tenure was already in place because of the existence of the Rural Family Medicine Residency Program that was established in 1994. The initial complement of community physicians committed to teaching had already been established and has continued to grow. The faculty is currently comprised of University-employed physicians, as well as physicians in community private practice, the VA system and a local Federally Qualified Healthcare Center (FQHC). Today, there are nearly 100 full-time and 75 adjunct part-time faculty.

WVU-Eastern was also created as a cooperative endeavor between WVU-SOM and the West Virginia School of Osteopathic Medicine (WVSOM), each sending students to the campus for their third and fourth clinical years.

Structure, Governance, and Funding:

The campus is led by the Associate Vice President of Health Sciences and Dean of WVU's Eastern Campus, who reports to the Vice President and Executive Dean at the Main Campus.

Two Student Services deans (an Associate and an Assistant) are responsible for student administrative and educational affairs as well as faculty development. These deans report to the Eastern Campus Dean, and receive guidance and support from counterparts at the Main Campus.

The primary source of funding for initial campus development was special appropriations from the state legislature. In 2002, a permanent line-item in the state budget was created for the Eastern Campus. Senator Robert C. Byrd procured special funding for the construction of a dedicated academic building in Martinsburg, West Virginia which houses the Dean's office, Student Services, student study and recreation areas, a large auditorium, several classrooms, a simulation lab, and administrative offices. Current campus operations are funded cooperatively from direct hospital support, the state budget, and the faculty practice plan.

Student Body:

There are 14 students from the WVU-SOM and six students from WVSOM in each of the third and fourth years. Students accepted to WVU-SOM are expected to review information on the three WVU campuses, and submit campus choice upon confirmation of their acceptance. Students are assigned based on choice until the 14 Eastern spots are filled. The first two basic science years are spent at the main campus, followed by the two clinical years at the Eastern Campus. Students on this campus can choose the same specialized tracks available on all three campuses — Global Health, Rural Medicine, and the newest track, Culinary and Lifestyle Medicine.

WVSOM (osteopathic) students submit their campus choice in the fall of their sophomore year, and six are selected by their school to attend during their clinical years.

Some students choose Eastern Campus because they are from the area or attended a pipeline program called MedSTEP at Shepherd University in the Eastern Panhandle. Others choose it for the unique curriculum or campus proximity to Maryland, Washington, D.C., or Virginia. Over the past 10 years, 119 students have graduated, entering 21 different specialties: 63 students in the primary care fields of Pediatrics, Family Medicine and Internal Medicine, 32 in surgical specialties, and 24 students in non-primary care/non-surgical fields (Anesthesia, Neurology, Pathology, ER, Psychiatry, etc). Residency location choices have included 35 students staying in West Virginia, 30 in the neighboring states of Pennsylvania, Virginia, and Maryland, and 54 students in 25 other states. Thirty-one former students have returned as faculty to the Eastern Campus, with 24 of them currently in practice and teaching in 2017.

Other learners on the campus include:

- Family Medicine Residents
- Visiting ENT and OB/GYN residents from WVU Main Campus
- Pharm D, DNP, PA, NP, Nurse midwife and Pathology Tech students
- Psychology (Psych D Residents)

The Family Medicine Residency with 18 residents is currently the only residency at the Eastern Campus. This allows the students to have close working relationships with the clinical faculty, with one-on-one teaching experiences in most venues. They have intra-professional educational experiences with mid-level practitioners such as PAs, NPs, nurse midwives, and doctoral pharmacy students.

Curriculum:

WVU Eastern Campus follows a Longitudinal Integrated Curriculum. The third year clinical curriculum is delivered in two modules, each delivered over six months. The Jacques module includes Family Medicine, Pediatrics, and OB/GYN, and the Nau module encompasses Surgery, Internal Medicine, Neurology, and Psychiatry. Students change clerkship responsibilities every week or two in each module. Students are encouraged to follow their patients from one specialty to another (for instance, from the surgeon's office to the internist for pre-op consultation, or from the Family Medicine clinic to the neurologist's office). One-on-one mentoring is a key learning concept here. The students receive clerkship grades mid-rotation and at the end of the year, similar to main campus students. Test scores on the shelf exams have been comparable across campuses.

Unique Features:

- Half-day weekly "continuity clinic" with a local family physician, while developing their own panel of patients to be followed throughout the year.

- Formal group educational experiences, including lecture and small group learning sessions, are offered weekly on Friday afternoons.

- Dedicated communication curriculum: four hours monthly with a simulated patient and SIM-Man technology, covering topics such as motivational interviewing, delivering bad news, adolescent interviewing, medical error prevention, child abuse awareness, and responsible "controlled medication" prescribing.

- Allopathic and osteopathic students training together in clinical rotations provides unique perspectives.

- Nutrition curriculum: Medical Student Curriculum in Healthy Eating, Exercise and Food Science (MedCHEFS), which includes two hours monthly of hands-on sessions in which students create a variety of foods, review case histories, and are mentored by a local chef.

- With few resident learners present, most faculty/student encounters are one-on-one teaching opportunities.

Accomplishments and Challenges:

Accomplishments

- **New Medical School Educational Track**

  The MedCHEFS curriculum has been active at Eastern Campus since 2012. In 2017, the Eastern faculty created a Culinary and Lifestyle Medicine Track, which was approved by LCME and began recruiting students in the August 2017-2018 cycle. The track will be administered by Eastern faculty, but students on any campus can participate.

- **Community Education**

  A Mini-Med School monthly two-hour series began in 2009, in which faculty, residents and/or students deliver history of medicine or factual medical anatomy or physiology lessons that can be clearly understood by an adult lay population. Topics have included stroke, obesity, vaccines, and new medical interventions.

Challenges

- Developing research and educational opportunities for the medical students and faculty to promote scholarly work, despite the challenges of a physician shortage.

Future Plans:

Short term goals

- Metabolic Center of Excellence
- Expanding both the primary care and specialty faculty
- Laying groundwork for an Internal Medicine residency
- New service lines for Neurosurgery and Orthopedics, developing a Vascular Institute and a Cancer Institute, and expanding pediatric specialty presence

Long term goals

- Building a Maternal/Pediatric Hospital
- Adding a Cardio-thoracic Surgery service line

26. Western University Schulich School of Medicine & Dentistry, Windsor Campus

Authors:

- Gerry Cooper, Ed.D.,
  Associate Dean, Windsor Campus,
  Associate Professor of Psychiatry,
  Schulich School of Medicine & Dentistry, Western University

- Mark Awuku MB, ChB, FRCP(C), FAAP, FGCP,
  Professor of Paediatrics,
  Schulich School of Medicine & Dentistry, Western University

Regional Campus:

Schulich School of Medicine & Dentistry – Windsor Campus
Location: Windsor, Ontario, Canada

Institution (main campus):

Schulich School of Medicine & Dentistry, Western University
Location: London, Ontario, Canada

History and Mission:

The Windsor Campus (WC) opened in September 2008 in response to a longstanding shortage of physicians. This medical education campus is a collaboration between two universities: Western University (Western), home to the Schulich School of Medicine and Dentistry, and the University of Windsor (UWindsor), which hosts Windsor's Regional Medical Campus (RMC). WC staff are employees of UWindsor. Western and UWindsor are roughly a two-hour drive apart. Windsor is Canada's southernmost city across the international border from Detroit, Michigan.

Medical students began training in Windsor in 2002 when several clinical clerks rotated for a few weeks at a time. Word quickly spread that there was great potential for medical training in this community. The number of learners and duration of training increased substantially, leading to the Windsor Campus' opening as a formal RMC six years later. Initially there were 24 year-one medical students, then 30 in 2009, and 38 each year afterwards. Today there are 152 students across four years of undergraduate medical education (UME) in this community. The WC is a vibrant RMC best described as a "combined model" (Cheifetz, McOwen and Gagne, 2014) with basic sciences/pre-clinical studies in the first two years followed by clinical training in years three and four.

In addition to medical students, WC supports a range of postgraduate training across a variety of specialties, including full-time trainees in Family Medicine (10 PGY-1, 10 PGY-2, and up to 4 PGY-3) and Psychiatry (this program began in 2016 and when fully implemented will have at least two residents in each of the PGY-1 through PGY-5 years). There are approximately 350 adjunct faculty members, the vast majority of whom are active physician clinicians. To date, the WC has graduated roughly 240 physicians and has been exceptionally welcomed by the local communities it serves, the urban city of Windsor and surrounding rural Essex County, with a total population of roughly 400,000.

Administratively there were some growing pains at the WC in its formative years; this resulted in an Acting Associate Dean for an extended period of time and an external review.

Structure, Governance and Funding:

A formal affiliation agreement exists between Western University and UWindsor. It was approved by each university president and was renewed in 2016 for a 10-year period. A governing committee chaired by the Dean has equal representation from both universities. WC's Associate Dean holds a faculty appointment at Western and belongs to decanal and executive teams within the Schulich School of Medicine, thus giving ample access to the Dean and other senior leaders within the School. The Associate Dean also serves as Director of Medical Studies at UWindsor, thus enabling supervisory responsibilities for the UWindsor administrative team at WC. An Assistant Dean for Windsor Faculty Affairs leads WC's recruitment, retention, and oversight of its professoriate. An operations manager and a clinical education team leader complete WC's administrative leadership team.

WC also has its own academic leadership structure including:

1. Academic Directors for each of the core specialties at each of the Undergraduate Medical Education (UME) and postgraduate levels

2. Course Coordinators for each of the pre-clinical courses within the UME curriculum

3. Clerkship & Electives Coordinator

It is expected that all of these Windsor Campus leaders regularly correspond and collaborate with their counterparts at Western's main campus.

WC funding is collected at and distributed by Western. Funding for Schulich School of Medicine and Dentistry arrives from a variety of sources, primarily grants from both government and research, as well as tuition and donations.

Student Body:

WC students are closely connected to their main campus counterparts. The admissions process is uniform and all students experience an orientation program (including a White Coat Ceremony) at the main campus. Afterwards, students initiate several cross-campus integration activities throughout the year. They pride themselves on remaining a cohesive group until graduation (also held at the main campus).

Students who have graduated from WC have been very successful within the Canadian residency match process (99.2 percent), although a few needed to enter round two. Most have matched into Family Medicine (49 percent), Internal Medicine (16 percent), and Surgery (9 percent).

There is also a growing cadre of full-time and visiting residents supported by WC. These trainees are invited to all special events and they are encouraged to participate in various teaching and scholarship activities.

Curriculum:

Schulich Medicine students share the same UME curriculum regardless of location, including a minimum of four weeks' training at a rural clinical site. In Windsor, most clinical instruction is located at two hospitals, Windsor Regional Hospital and Hôtel-Dieu Grace Healthcare, as well as a variety of community-based clinics. Assessment protocols are identical at each campus. Currently, the curriculum is undergoing an intensive competency-based medical education (CBME) renewal. The UME Associate Dean is the School's Chief Academic Officer and the WC Associate Dean will substitute as required. Medical Student Performance Reviews (MSPR) are written by the UME Associate Dean.

The Learner Equity and Wellness (LEW) team at Schulich School of Medicine and Dentistry oversees student health and includes personnel located at WC. Communications across the campuses are seamless, utilizing electronic communications, video-conferencing, and telephone augmented by periodic in-person meetings.

Unique Characteristics:

WC students often cite increased hands-on training as an advantage of the regional campus. Clerkship rotations at WC are consistently rated very highly. Initially, students felt disadvantaged by having too few research opportunities at WC. However, a unique program known as **SWORP** (**S**chulich **W**indsor **O**pportunities for **R**esearch Excellence **P**rogram), jointly funded by Western and UWindsor now provides for WC students to engage in summer research projects.

Visiting students and residents are housed at the state-of-the-art Medical Arts Building[2] which also acts as a potential recruitment strategy for the local community.

Proximity of the WC to UWindsor's Faculty of Nursing has resulted in some wonderful collaborations, resource sharing, and ultimately, interprofessional educational opportunities (IPE). The fact that UWindsor's president attends Schulich Medicine's convocations alongside Western University's president speaks to the rich collaboration.

The strong commitment by local physicians to medical education is impressive. Their customary academic rank of adjunct professor remains a work in progress; nevertheless, they are passionate about broadly supporting the WC. This goes beyond teaching to include student bursaries via the Essex County Medical Society.

Accomplishments and Challenges:

Signature events like September's "Meet and Greet Event" and April's "Awards of Excellence Banquet", jointly celebrate a WC awards program and recognizes the students who are soon to graduate. While these initiatives have taken time to develop, it has been worth the effort. These events greatly foster familial-style collegiality, confidence, and excellence. They also serve to reinforce strong connections to the communities we serve. WC stories are also shared via an electronic newsletter (see online at: **http://www.schulich.uwo.ca/communications/windsor_newsletter/index.html**).

Fiscal restraint is ever present these days and thus an ongoing challenge. Occasionally, effort has been required to maintain a shared vision at both the main campus and WC, which is not surprising when considering diminishing resources. These instances, although infrequent, can require special diplomacy and sensitivity.

Future Plans:

The continued development of research opportunities remains a priority across the entire Winsor Campus, for both faculty and learners. We carefully monitor faculty engagement on a continual basis and this will remain a priority at the WC. Our geographical proximity to the U.S. also has us excited in regard to possible new partnerships and innovations in a cross-border context.

References:

1. Cheifetz, C., McOwen, K. & Gagné. (2014). Regional Medical Campuses: A New Classification System. Academic Medicine. 89(8): 1140-43.

2. Cooper, G., Sbrocca, N. & Vasapolli, B. (April, 2017). Physician recruitment to a RMC community via housing for visiting trainees. Paper presented at the 2017 Group on Regional Medical Campuses Spring Meeting, Orlando, Florida.

SECTION 3

Images from Regional Medical Campuses in the U.S. and Canada*

1. Campus of the University of Montreal in Mauricie [Campus de l'UdeM en Mauricie, Université de Montréal] (Trois-Rivières, Province de Québec, Canada)

Photo acknowledgement: Submitted by Pierre Gagné, M.D., FRCP(C), MSc

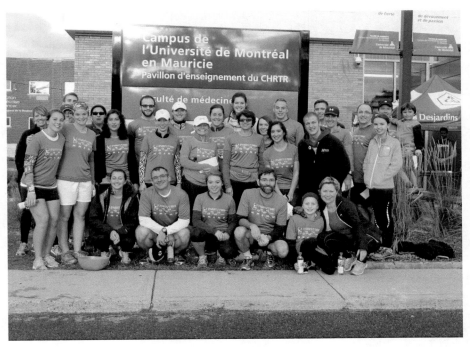

Mauricie Students Relay Marathon

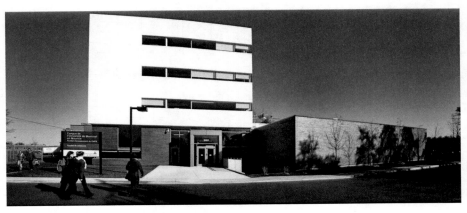

Campus of the University of Montreal in Mauricie

2. Des Moines Branch Campus, University of Iowa Carver College of Medicine *(Des Moines, Iowa)*

*Photo acknowledgement: Submitted by Steven R. Craig, M.D.

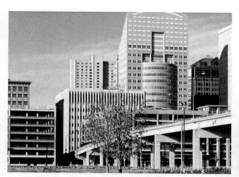

The Branch Campus is located on the western edge of downtown Des Moines

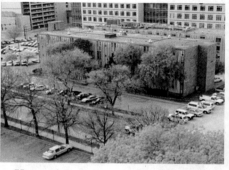

View of the Inntowner Apartments, Des Moines Branch Campus student housing facility

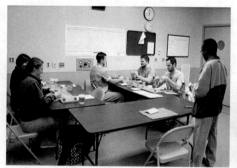

Des Moines Branch Campus surgery clerkship students work on knot tying in the Surgery Skills Lab on campus

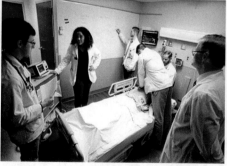

Core clerkship students completing team-based acute care simulation in the Dorner-Villeneuve Simulation Center at the Des Moines Branch Campus

3. Indiana University School of Medicine Bloomington (Bloomington, Indiana)

*Photo acknowledgement: Submitted by Peter M. Nalin, M.D.

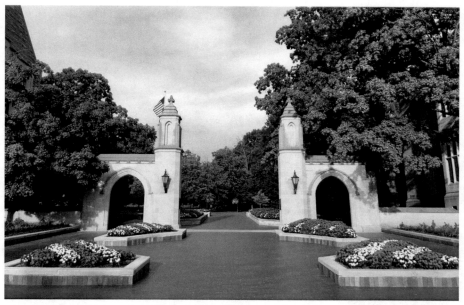

Indiana University, Bloomington (Photo credit: Peter M. Nalin, M.D.)

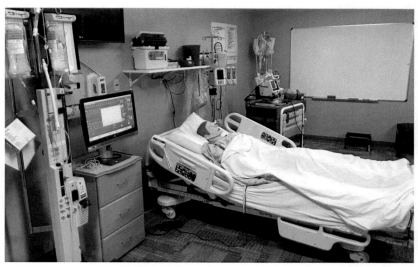

Indiana University School of Medicine Simulation Center
(Photo credit: Peter M. Nalin, M.D.)

4. Medical College of Georgia, Southeast Regional Campus *(Brunswick and Savannah, Georgia)*

Photo acknowledgement:
Submitted by Turner W. Rentz, Jr., M.D. and Frances Purcell, Ph.D

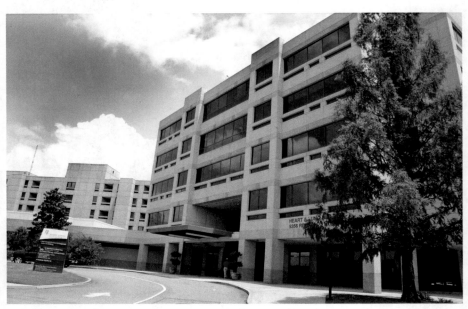

Saint Joseph's Hospital, Candler Health System, Savannah, GA

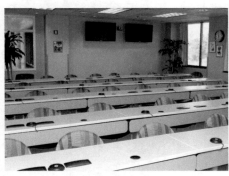

Classroom at
Medical College of Georgia

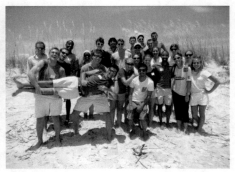

Medical College of Georgia
students

5. Medical College of Wisconsin-Central Wisconsin (*Wausau, Wisconsin*)

*Photo acknowledgement: Submitted by Lisa Grill Dodson, M.D.

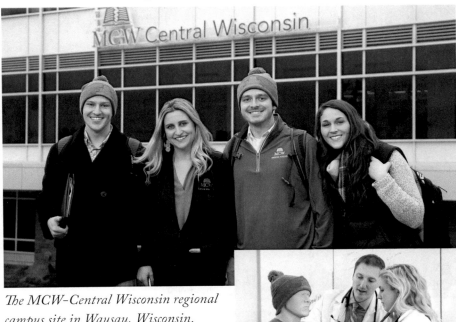

The MCW-Central Wisconsin regional campus site in Wausau, Wisconsin. Class of 2019 students

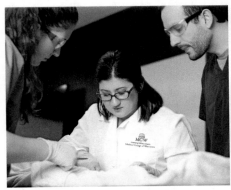

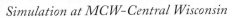

Simulation at MCW-Central Wisconsin

Students in lab at the MCW-Central Wisconsin

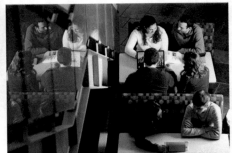

Students at MCW-Central Wisconsin gather for a study session

6. Mercer University School of Medicine, Columbus Campus *(Columbus, Georgia)*

*Photo acknowledgement: Submitted by Alice Aumann House, M.D.

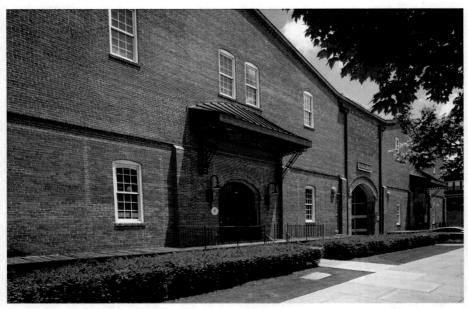

Columbus Campus New Entrance (Photo credit: John Knight)

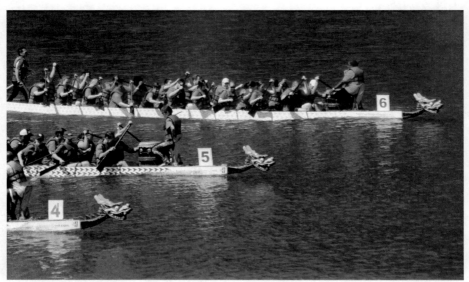

Dragon Boat Race (Photo credit: Kristen Kettlehut)

7. Northern Medical Program, University of British Columbia *(University of Northern British Columbia, Prince George, British Columbia, Canada)*

*Photo acknowledgement: Submitted by Sean B. Maurice, Ph.D. and Paul J. Winwood, MB, BS, DM, FRCPC

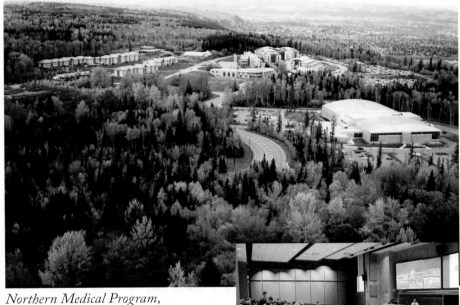

Northern Medical Program, University of British Columbia (Photo credit: Courtesy of UNBC)

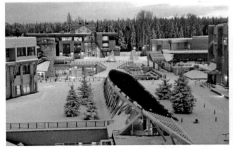

Northern Medical Program, University of British Columbia (Photo credit: Courtesy of UNBC)

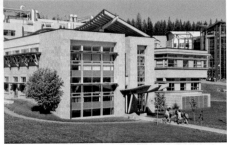

(Photo credit: Sonya Kruger, NMP)

(Photo credit: Sonya Kruger, NMP)

8. Penn State College of Medicine, University Park Campus *(State College, Pennsylvania)*

*Photo acknowledgement: Submitted by Michael P. Flanagan, M.D.

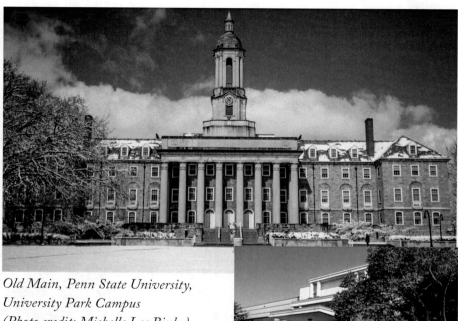

Old Main, Penn State University, University Park Campus (Photo credit: Michelle Lee Bixby)

Centre Medical Sciences Building, site of Student Learning Center, University Park Campus (Photo credit: Abby Drey)

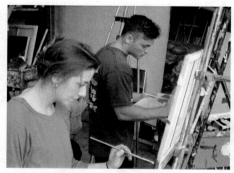

Medical Humanities Class, "Impressionism and the Art of Medical Communication", with MS IV students, University Park Campus (Photo credit: Michael Flanagan, M.D.)

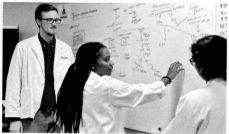

Inquiry Group with MS I students, Penn State College of Medicine, University Park Campus (Photo credit: Abby Drey)

9. Temple/St. Luke's School of Medicine (Bethlehem, Pennsylvania)

Photo acknowledgement:
Submitted by Joel C. Rosenfeld M.D., M.Ed. and Kathleen A. Dave, Ph.D.

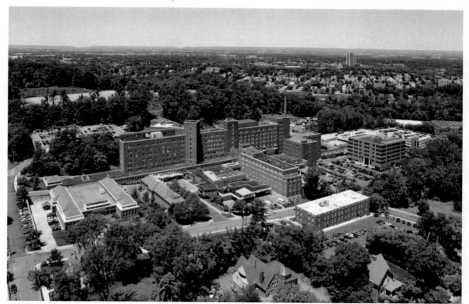

Temple/ St. Lukes School of Medicine Campus

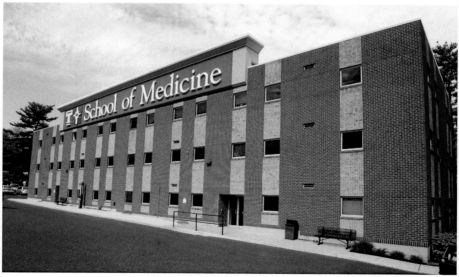

Temple/ St. Lukes School of Medicine

10. Texas Tech University Health Sciences Center School of Medicine, Permian Basin *(Odessa, Texas)*

*Photo acknowledgement: Submitted by Valerie Bauer, M.D.

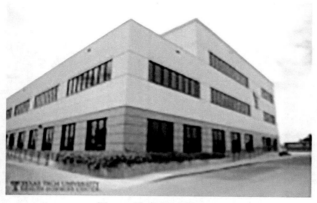

Texas Tech University
Health Sciences Center School of Medicine,
Permian Basin

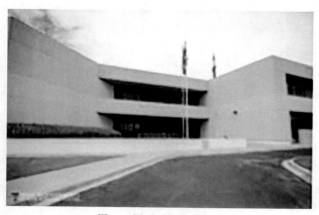

Texas Tech University
Health Sciences Center School of Medicine,
Permian Basin

11. Tufts University School of Medicine Maine Medical Center Program *(Portland, Maine)*

*Image acknowledgement: Submitted by Jo Ellen Linder, M.D.

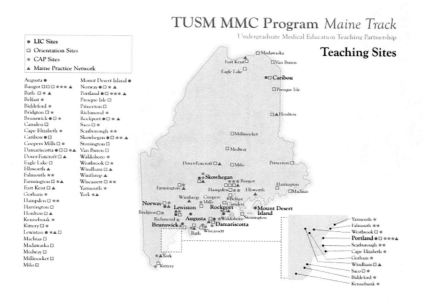

Teaching sites in Maine for the Tufts University School of Medicine Maine Track

12. UCSF Fresno Medical Education Program (Fresno, California)

*Photo acknowledgement: Submitted by Kenny Banh, M.D.

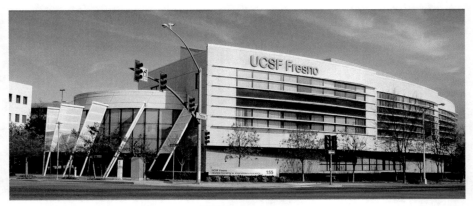

UCSF Fresno

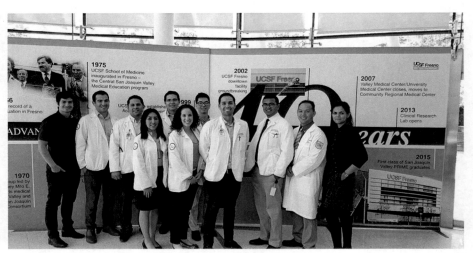

San Joaquin Valley PRIME Class of 2018

13. University of Alabama at Birmingham, Huntsville Regional Medical Campus *(Huntsville, Alabama)*

*Photo acknowledgement: Submitted by Lanita S. Carter, Ph.D.

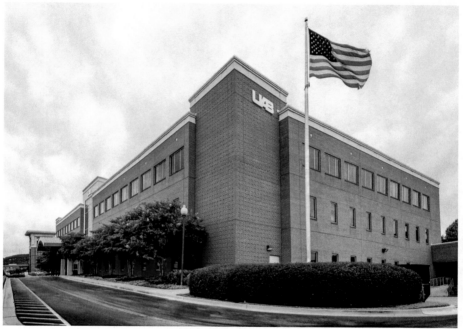

UAB Huntsville RMC

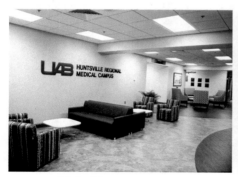

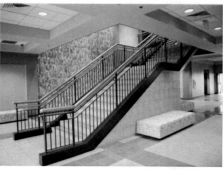

UAB Huntsville RMC
Third Floor Public Area

UAB Huntsville RMC
First Floor Lobby

14. University of Kansas School of Medicine-Salina (Salina, Kansas)

*Photo acknowledgement: Submitted by William Cathcart-Rake, M.D.

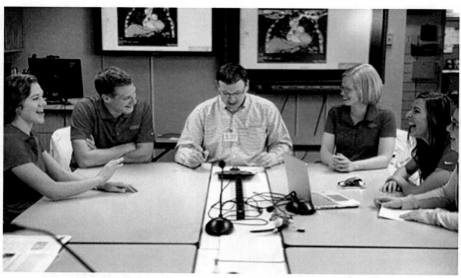

KUSM classroom instruction with students
(Photo credit: Garett S. Gabriel)

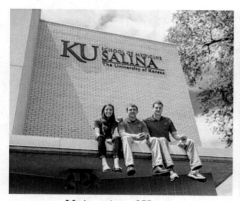

University of Kansas
School of Medicine-Salina
Campus Building
(Photo credit:
Garett S. Gabriel)

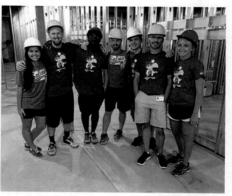

Members of the Class of 2021 in
new medical education building
under construction.
(Photo credit:
William Cathcart-Rake, M.D.)

15. University of Kentucky College of Medicine Rural Physician Leadership Program *(Morehead, Kentucky)*

*Photo acknowledgement: Submitted by Anthony Weaver M.D.

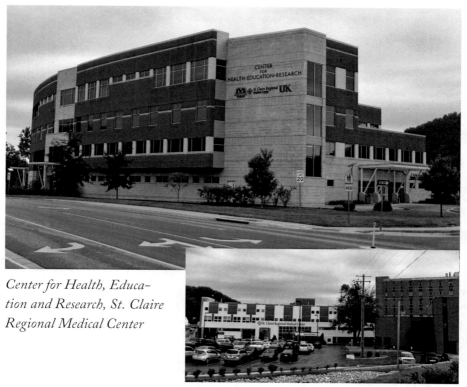

Center for Health, Education and Research, St. Claire Regional Medical Center

St. Claire Regional Medical Center

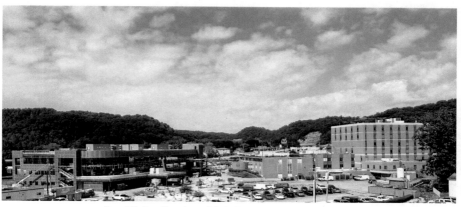

St. Claire Regional Medical Center expansion

16. University of Massachusetts Medical School - Baystate *(Springfield, Massachusetts)*

*Photo acknowledgement: Submitted by Rebecca D. Blanchard, Ph.D.

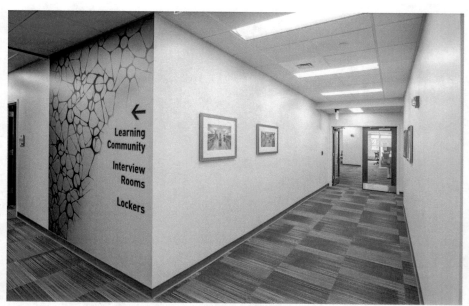

University of Massachusetts Medical School –Baystate

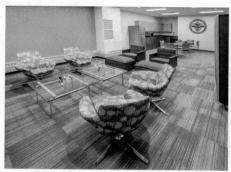

University of Massachusetts Medical School –Baystate

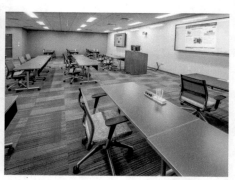

University of Massachusetts Medical School –Baystate

17. University of Minnesota Medical School, Duluth Campus *(Duluth, Minnesota)*

*Photo acknowledgement: Submitted by Paula M. Termuhlen, M.D.

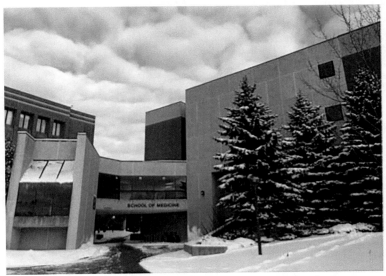

University of Minnesota Medical School, Duluth Campus
(Photo credit: Paula M. Termuhlen, M.D.)

18. University of South Dakota
Sanford School of Medicine *(State of South Dakota)*

Photo and image acknowledgement:
Submitted by Mark Beard, M.D., MHA and Shane Schellpfeffer, Ed.D.

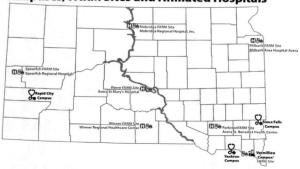

University of South Dakota Sanford School of Medicine campuses, FARM sites and affiliated hospitals.

Table 1: *Distance between Sanford School of Medicine sites*

Note: Calculated distances are driving distances.

	Sioux Falls		Rapid City		Yankton		Vermillion		Milbank		Mobridge		Parkston		Pierre		Spearfish	
	mi	km	mi	km	mi	km	mi	km	mi	km	mi	km	mi	km	mi	km	mi	km
Rapid City	347	558																
Yankton	79	127	356	573														
Vermillion	62	100	390	628	27	43												
Milbank	126	203	458	737	201	323	184	296										
Mobridge	307	494	233	375	324	521	364	586	200	322								
Parkston	74	119	296	476	61	98	88	142	203	327	264	425						
Pierre	225	362	172	277	234	377	268	431	234	377	111	179	174	280				
Spearfish	393	632	49	79	401	645	437	703	413	665	223	359	341	549	194	312		
Winner	169	272	215	346	146	235	173	278	301	484	202	325	97	156	94	151	261	420

Driving distance between Sanford School of Medicine sites

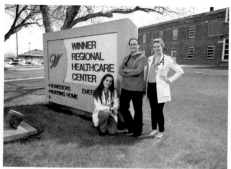

Winner Regional Healthcare Center

19. Washington State University, Elson S. Floyd College of Medicine
(Four Regional Clinical Campuses: Everett, Vancouver, Tri-Cities, and Spokane, Washington)

Photo acknowledgement: Submitted by Ralitsa Akins, M.D., Ph.D.

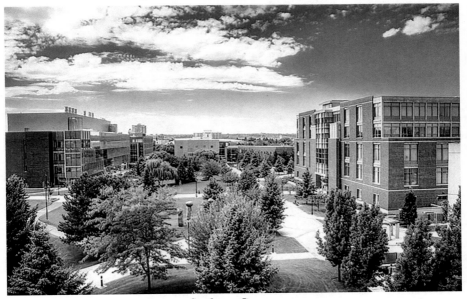

Spokane Campus

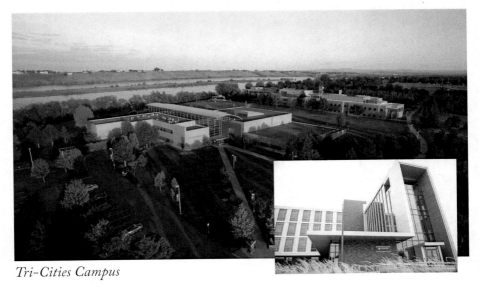

Tri-Cities Campus

20. Western University Schulich School of Medicine & Dentistry, Windsor Campus (Windsor, Ontario, Canada)

*Photo acknowledgement: Submitted by Gerry Cooper Ed.D.

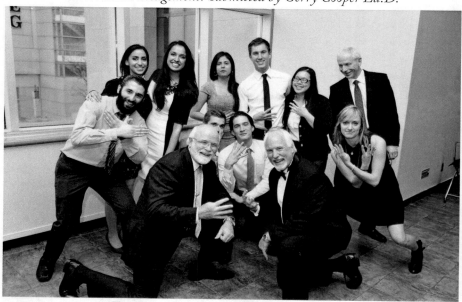

Faculty and students of Western University
Schulich School of Medicine & Dentistry, Windsor Campus

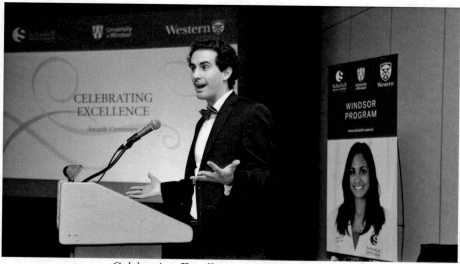

Celebrating Excellence at Windsor Campus

Afterword

In the foreword to this book, E. Eugene Marsh, M.D. shares what people often say when describing medical school regional campuses: "If you've seen one regional campus, you've seen one regional campus". While this may be true, there are also several questions that, when answered individually, give a picture of each regional campus, and when taken collectively, demonstrate important commonalities among these campuses. These questions are:

- **What is the purpose of the campus, and why was it begun?** Was the purpose to expand the size of the medical school, to involve a new geographic region, or both? Was the school intended to focus on primary care?

- **What is the structure of the campus?** Does it include the preclinical years of medical school, the clinical years, or both, and is Graduate Medical Education (GME) present on campus? Are other programs involved, such as Physician Assistant or Nurse Practitioner training programs?

- **How is the campus funded?** What is the mix of state appropriation, tuition, grants, contracts, and philanthropic dollars included in the budget?

- **How are accreditation issues handled?** Does the campus have separate LCME accreditation status, or is it a track within the main campus's system? Does the campus have its own ACGME institutional accreditation?

- **Does the campus own or manage a health delivery system?** Are there university-owned medical practices, clinics, or other practice sites involved, or are other sites involved in education?

- **What hospital systems are involved with the education of learners?** Who owns these systems? What type of voice does the university have within the systems? What effect, if any, have hospital mergers, acquisitions and other transformations had on the educational programs?

- **What is the nature of the faculty?** Are faculty members full-time, part time, employed by the university, employed by others, or volunteer? How is this mix changing?

- **What is the overall capacity for education on the campus?** This includes the physical capacity, including lecture and conference rooms, study space, and the human resource capacity for providing sufficient clinical rotations for learners. The combination of physician and human capacities must provide for a rich and varied learning environment and a large enough "practice field" for all involved learners. If volunteer faculty members are involved, how are they sustained?

- **What is the learning environment?** Given the diverse nature of the faculty and environmental structures, how are program requirements maintained? How are issues of professionalism and the "hidden curriculum" managed?

- **What type of curriculum is in place?** Is a block curriculum used, or longitudinal rotations, or both?

The answers to these questions often interact in interesting ways as a campus develops and matures. There may be conflicts between the original mission of the campus and reality based factors that cause modifications to campus structure and function. For example, at the University of Oklahoma-Tulsa (OU-TU) School of Community Medicine in Tulsa, it was originally hoped by many stakeholders that an independent four-year medical school would be formed within northeastern Oklahoma. Major philanthropic gifts were donated with this concept in mind. However, this structure was eventually judged to not be feasible due to total cost. A new structure emerged, with Tulsa continuing as a clinical campus for the University of Oklahoma College of Medicine, and the University of Tulsa assisting in areas of basic science education. In addition, the clinical campus expanded from a two-year to a full four-year medical school site. The campus now also includes 15 residency/fellowship programs and a set of university-owned practice sites with more than 250,000 visits each year.

This book is a major step forward in describing the structure and function of regional medical campuses. We are in a time of relative turbulence in the United States health care system, with frequent regional consolidations, the development of value-based compensation systems and a significant physician shortage expected in the next decade. Regional medical campuses can provide their parent universities with much needed flexibilities to successfully meet these challenges. In addition, such campuses provide a location for innovation in areas such as primary care, curriculum development, and collaborative learning. Demonstrated success in these areas can be diffused to other schools and campuses through the sharing of creative ideas, solutions to common challenges and evidenced-based results. This book provides exactly that. As such, it is an important new resource for all those interested in regional medical campuses, whether they be well-established, in development, or under consideration.

James M. Herman, M.D. M.S.P.H.

Dean, Professor, and Morningcrest Endowed Leadership Chair
The University of Oklahoma
OU–TU School of Community Medicine
Tulsa, Oklahoma

Index

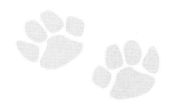
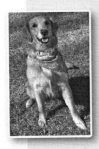
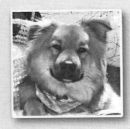
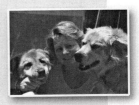

Over the years, we have adopted a number of dogs from rescues and shelters. First there was Bear and after he passed, Ginger and Scout. Now, we have Kira, another rescue. They have brought immense joy and love not just into our lives, but into the lives of all who met them.

We want you to know a portion of the profits of this book will be donated in Bear, Ginger and Scout's memory to local animal shelters, parks, conservation organizations, and other individuals and nonprofit organizations in need of assistance.

— Douglas & Sherri Brown,
President & Vice-President of Atlantic Publishing

Faculty Editor Biographies

Michael P. Flanagan, M.D., FAAFP is a Professor of Family and Community Medicine at the Penn State College of Medicine. He serves as Assistant Dean for Student Affairs, Vice-Chair for Family Medicine and medical director at the University Park Campus in State College, Pennsylvania.

❦❦❦❦❦❦

Kristen M. Grine, D.O. is an Assistant Professor of Family and Community Medicine and serves as a medical director and Co-Clerkship Director of Family Medicine at the Penn State College of Medicine University Park Campus.

❦❦❦❦❦❦

Christopher R. Heron, M.D. is a core faculty member for the Penn State Health Family and Community Medicine Residency at Mount Nittany Medical Center in State College, Pennsylvania. He is an Assistant Professor of Family and Community Medicine, and also serves as Director of Clinical Information Technology at the University Park Campus.

❦❦❦❦❦❦

E. Eugene Marsh, M.D. is the former founding Senior Associate Dean and master educator at the Penn State College of Medicine University Park Campus. Now retired, he continues to serve as a Clinical Professor of Neurology.

Mark B. Stephens, M.D., MS, FAAFP is a Professor of Family and Community Medicine at the Penn State College of Medicine. He also serves as Clinical Course Director for first year students, Co-Clerkship Director of Family Medicine and Associate Vice-Chair for Research at the University Park Campus.

Jeffrey G. Wong, M.D. is the Associate Dean for Education and a Professor of Medicine at the Penn State College of Medicine University Park Campus.